Epidemiology of Injuries in Sports

Gian Luigi Canata • Henrique Jones
Editors

Epidemiology of Injuries in Sports

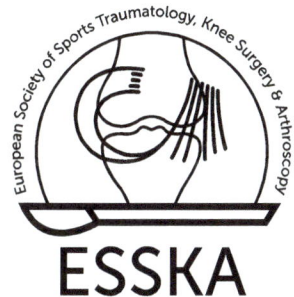

ESSKA

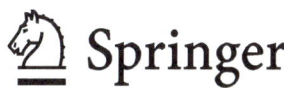

Editors
Gian Luigi Canata
Centre of Sports Traumatology
Koelliker Hospital
TORINO, Italy

Henrique Jones
Orthopedic and Sports Medicine Clinic
Montijo, Portugal

ISBN 978-3-662-64531-4   ISBN 978-3-662-64532-1   (eBook)
https://doi.org/10.1007/978-3-662-64532-1

This Springer imprint is published by the registered company Springer-Verlag GmbH, DE part of Springer Nature.
The registered company address is: Heidelberger Platz 3, 14197 Berlin, Germany

Preface

This booklet presents an update on the epidemiology of injuries in 24 different sports.

ESMA-ESSKA is dedicated to sports medicine and its mission includes the prevention of injuries.

New epidemiological information could be a useful tool helping to improve our preventive measures.

We are grateful to the authors for their outstanding contribution and for the time they dedicated to this project.

ESSKA must be commended for the full unconditioned support that has made possible the production of this publication that in our aim will be a professional support to all those involved in Sports Traumatology.

TORINO, Italy   Gian Luigi Canata
Montijo, Portugal   Henrique Jones

Contents

Archery

1

Fiammetta Scarzella

1.1 Characteristics of the Sport

Archery is an ancient skill, first applied in hunting and warfare, with an early progression towards a competitive sport. The first known organized competition was held in England in 1583. Archery first appeared in Olympic Games in 1900 and was contested again in 1904, 1908 and 1920 and then re-introduced in 1972; the team competition was added in Seoul in 1988. Nowadays, archery includes a wide range of different disciplines, among which only the recurve bow represents an Olympic discipline. The barebow consists of a riser with a handle, two doubles shaped limbs and a bowstring; if you add a sight, stabilization bars and the clicker you get the recurve bow. A compound bow is a bow that uses a levering system of cables and pulleys to bend the limbs; this system grants the user a mechanical advantage, and so the limbs of a compound bow are much stiffer than those of a recurve bow; additionally, magnifying sight, stabilizers, rear peep sights and mechanical release devices are used to increase the level of consistency and accuracy [1].

A sport bow weighs approximately 2–3 kg, and the drawing weight ranges between 35 lbs to 45 lbs for recurve and barebow archers and from 50 lbs to 60 lbs for compound archers. During a competition, archers shoot from 36 to 144 arrows a day depending on the type of competition; the target can be at the distance of 18 m for indoor competition or up to the distance of 90 m for outdoor competition. The Olympic competition takes place at a distance of 70 m.

1.2 Physiological and Biomechanical Demands on Athletes

Archery is a highly isometric sport, which requires strength and endurance of the upper body, the arms and shoulder girdle. It can be classified as a fine motor skill. Good body posture and balance are also essential requirements in successful shooting movement in archery. The shot can be divided into phases: hold the bow, drawing phase, final draw, aiming and release. Firstly, the arm nocks the arrow onto the string and hold the string with three fingers (ring, middle and index) of the drawing hand (or with the mechanical release regarding the compound bow); the bow arm is raised and the bow is held in the direction of the target; simultaneously, the drawing arm is extended to 90°; the drawing arm now exerts a dynamic pulling movement until the release is executed. The shot is completed by the follow-through.

F. Scarzella (✉)
Istituto di Medicina dello Sport, Torino, Italy
e-mail: fiammetta.scarzella@imsto.it

© The Author(s), under exclusive license to Springer-Verlag GmbH, DE, part of Springer Nature 2022
G. L. Canata, H. Jones (eds.), *Epidemiology of Injuries in Sports*,
https://doi.org/10.1007/978-3-662-64532-1_1

Maintaining the appropriate stance and the consistency of the stance from shot to shot is essential to improve performance in archery. Postural muscles contract isometrically to maintain correct stance and balance. Upright position of the spine against gravity is maintained by isometric contraction of extensor muscles of the trunk: erector spine, deep posterior spinal muscles and semispinal muscles. Flexor muscles of the trunk (rectus abdominis, oblique externus abdominis and obliques internus abdominis) also contract isometrically against the pulling effect of trunk extensor muscles to prevent hyperextension at the trunk, especially during the release phase. The balance of muscle strength between trunk flexor and extensor is important in preventing sway of the body and maintaining correct body posture and equilibrium without excessive effort or tension during the shooting movement.

During drawing, anchoring, releasing and follow-through phases, rotation to the target of the neck is maintained by isometric contraction, while during the execution of the rotation movement, muscles contract concentrically; the muscles involved are sternocleidomastoid, suboccipitalis, cervical and capital portions of erector spine, semispinalis and deep posterior spinal muscles.

Archery requires one arm pulling the bowstring while pushing the bow with the other arm. The pushing arm is called the bow arm and the pulling arm, the draw arm. Although they have opposite functions, most of the joint positions are similar. The main anatomic position of both the bow and the draw arm is composed of horizontal extension and abduction of humerus at the glenohumeral joint accompanied by scapular adduction at the shoulder girdle. There is forearm extension at the elbow joint of the bow arm, while flexion is maintained in the bow arm. As the bow arm is raised to shoulder height sideward to the target, the scapula gets closer to the spine. Rhomboids major and minor, second and third parts of trapezius are involved in scapular adduction which stabilized scapula. These muscles contract concentrically during the execution of the movement and then they contract isometrically to maintain this position throughout the shooting. In the draw arm, a strong concentric contraction of the scapular adductor muscles is required during the drawing action. After that, these muscles contract isometrically to keep this position throughout the shooting movement. Then upward rotation of the scapula, which is performed by serratus anterior and the lower fibres of trapezius, enables the head of the humerus to be accommodated at the shoulder joint. In order to stabilize the scapula trough, the shooting movement strength and endurance of the shoulder girdle muscles should be sufficient. Abduction of the upper arm also results in scapular upward rotation, which is attained by contraction of the serratus anterior and lower fibres of the trapezius. The glenohumeral joint provides stability of the shoulder joint and is the key to accurate shooting. Abduction at the glenohumeral joint is achieved by contraction of the deltoid and supraspinatus; horizontal extension at the glenohumeral joint is accomplished by the contraction of the posterior part of the deltoid, infraspinatus and teres minor. At the beginning of the movement, muscles contract concentrically to perform the related movement, and they contract isometrically to maintain the position. Because an archer is required to perform many shootings during both training and competition, these muscles should have enough strength and endurance to prevent fatigue and accuracy reduction of the movement. There is also an internal rotation at the glenohumeral joint which is performed by the contraction of the anterior part of the deltoid, pectoralis major, latissimus dorsi, teres major and subscapularis. In the draw arm, pulling the bowstring towards the anchor point is accomplished by horizontal extension at the glenohumeral joint combined with the contraction of scapular adductor muscles (posterior portion of the deltoid, subscapularis, infraspinatus and latissimus dorsi). The elbow joint of the bow arm is in the extension and semipronation position. Triceps brachii and anconeus are involved isometrically to maintain the extension position at the elbow joint, which enables the bow arm to resist the pressure of the bow. Semipronation of the elbow is maintained by isometric contraction of the pronator teres and pronator quadratus. The elbow joint in the draw arm is in flexion position; biceps brachii, brachioradialis and brachialis are involved. Slight extension position is maintained at the radiocarpal joint of the bow hand to keep the wrist in functional anatomical position. Isometric contraction of wrist flexor muscles, flexor carpi ulnaris and flexor carpi radialis aids to resist the pressure of the bow by keeping the functional anatomic position of the wrist and preventing greater extension. The hand should be in a relaxed, comfortable position and the bow should not be held or griped. In the draw wrist, a neutral slight extension position is maintained at the radiocarpal joint to keep the wrist in functional anatomical position. Extensor carpi radialis brevis and lungus and extensor carpi ulnaris are involved. Because in the draw arm the dorsal surface of the hand is kept as flat as possible, metacarpophalangeal joints are in extension. The extensor digitorum, extensor indicis and extensor digiti minimi muscles are involved in this movement. The bowstring is placed on the distal interphalangeal joints of index, middle and ring fingers and held by the flexion of these joints. Holding the bowstring requires flexion movement at both distal and proximal interphalangeal joints, which is attained by the contraction of flexor digitorum profundus and superficialis. The arrow is released by either the relaxation of the finger flexor muscles or concentric contraction of finger extensor muscles or a combination of these two movements.

Some studies [2] using electromyography (EMG) to investigate muscular activation noted that the better an archer is, the lower the muscle activity that is used. It is common that lower level archers do use much more muscle activity in muscle groups which should not be involved in archery. Archers who are tense and/or use more muscle activity than needed can easily be injured. One of the reasons is that archers who are tense need more activity in the muscles involved in pulling because the activity has to overcome the tension to get the arm moving. Nishizono et al. conducted a study to analyse the activation levels of muscle groups involved in archery shooting. The muscular contraction level was higher in back muscles than in arm muscles in world-class

archers compared with middle class and beginner archers. In addition, the world-class archers displayed almost the same level of activity in back muscles on both sides. The beginner and middle-class archers showed an unbalanced activity in the same muscle groups. The release phase must be well balanced and highly reproducible. Therefore, the balance between the contraction levels of the back muscles in both sides can be used as an indicator of performance level. The drawing arm force needs to be equal to the force of the bow arm muscles so that the release of the bowstring by the drawing arm will not disturb the statical position of the extended bow arm.

1.3   Epidemiology of Injuries

Archery is known as a low risk sport. In the FITA study of 2002, the relative injury incidence per 1000 training hours is 0.2 for senior archers and 0.6 for junior archers. Female archers seem to be more prone to injuries than males. Shoulder was the most injured site (49%) followed by fingers (12.3%) and elbow (11.4) in senior archers, while among junior archers fingers were the most injured site (37.5%) followed by shoulder (26.8%) and spine (16.1%). More than 70% of all injuries were found to be related to upper extremities among senior; 82% among juniors. The majority (79.2% among senior, 62% among juniors) had a chronic problem [3].

Overuse injuries are mainly located in the shoulder region, especially in the drawing shoulder [4]. The second most common overuse injury is in the bow arm. Caused by asymmetrical loads, overuse can be found at typical unilateral localization. Overuse injuries are mainly injuries of tendons, ligaments and joints. Presently available literature reports excessive drawing weigh or number of arrow shot during training, lack of strength, lack of warm-up before training sessions and competitions, and incorrect technique (or a change in shooting technique) as risk factors for overuse injuries. Repetitive raising of the bow arm and drawing arm as well as drawing movement is capable of causing impingement in both arms but mainly in the bow arm. A common fault associated with impingement syndromes in athletes is poor scapular stabilization. The shoulder girdle is then not anchored or positioned correctly putting the subacromial structures at high risk for impingement. The muscles of the bow arm are less often injured but also can be subject to repetitive strain if the scapula is not strong and stable. Without the rhomboids and lower/middle trapezius muscles securing the scapula to the rib cage, the entire shoulder complex is elevated when the strong deltoid group contract. Especially, the sovraspinatus and long biceps tendons as well as bursa subacromialis are compressed under the acromion. This causes inflammation such as tendinosis and bursitis, which cause pain. The FITA study of 2002 stated that overuse injuries were located mainly in the shoulder (46%). Tendinosis or impingement represented 60.5% of the overuse injuries. Mann [5] also described overuse of the drawing shoulder as the most common overuse injury in archers. He stated that less strength in female archers caused higher numbers of overuse injuries among female participants in his study. A lack of strength combined with earlier exhaustion and deficiencies in execution are possibly the reason for high number of overuse injuries. Less trained athletes will get tired in their stabilizing trunk muscles first; then the upper body tilts towards the bow. This changes the direct lineforce transmission from the stretched arm to the shoulder girdle to a nonlinear transmission: the shoulder girdle follows the trunk and dives at the bow arm side, a move which is compensated by elevation of the bow arm. This causes narrowing of the subacromial space and therefore increases the pressure to all structures with the consequence of impingement. Repetitive micro trauma caused by the typical movement of the archer is seen as the underlying cause of acromioclavicular joint arthrosis that represents rare overuse injuries in archery. In the FITA study, 11.4% of overuse injuries were found in the elbow. Predominantly, lateral epicondylitis was reported, which is caused by repetitive turning and stretching movements of the forearm. A faulty position and exerting strenuous traction when pulling arrows from too densely packed target butts have been found to be

the most frequent cause of the onset of epitrochleitis in the drawing arm. Infrequent localizations of overuse injuries were hand and fingers. Here, tendosynovitis was found most frequently. Repetitive movements with loads, as well as vibrations of the bow handle during the shot can be the reason. Approximately 10% of the archers surveyed by the FITA Medical Committee listed back pain as one of their injuries.

Acute injuries are usually caused by material failure (fracture of bow, arrow and string during the shot) or by the string touching the bow arm. They include hematomas and wounds. Haematoma of the forearm affects mainly the novice and beginners and stems from a poor position of the bow arm.

Compared to other sports, archery has a very low injury risk. Acute injuries are particularly rare in professional archers.

In our experience, one of the most frequently occurring clinical manifestations among archers is dorsalgia and interscapular pain irradiated at the mid-dorsal level, with an increase in pain with increasing workloads. The reasons for this pain are to be found in a series of causes that lead to a dysfunction of the muscles of the dorsal and intersapular district. In most cases, scapula pain is linked to muscle contractures, especially in the elevator scapulae; contractures can originate from trauma, excessive mechanical stress (exercises with weights) or from problems to the cervical spine (incorrect posture, herniated disc). The pain originates at the level of the upper margin of the scapula and can extend to the nuchal ligament in the central region of the cervical spine. Other typical manifestations are stiffness and reduction of shoulder's ROM. In the presence of concomitant problems of the cervical spine, there is irradiation of pain in the posteroanterior direction at the occipital level (musculotensive headaches). As regards the diagnostic procedure, the physical examination with a careful evaluation of the painful area and of the patient's history remains the main evaluation element. If problems are suspected in the cervical spine, instrumental investigations (radiography, magnetic resonance imaging) will be used, but it is always essential to exclude diseases affecting visceral structures or diseases of rheumatic origin.

1.4 Rehabilitation and Return to Play

The majority of the injuries are minor to moderate with a low rate of surgical intervention (6.7% among senior archers, 2.4% among junior archers).

One of the goals of sports medicine is to get the injured athlete back into the game as soon as possible without putting that individual at risk. After a musculoskeletal injury, the time for an athlete's recovery and return to play cannot be easily defined because these endpoints are affected by many factors, including the athlete's pre-injury condition, the type of tissue injured, the response to treatment, the need for surgical intervention and the psychological impact of the injury. Additionally, the individual athlete's motivation and/or any external pressure for performance must be considered. Overuse syndromes, re-injury and even long-term disability may occur when athletes return to play before adequate recovery. Successful return to play can be achieved by combining the principles of musculoskeletal care with an organized and multidisciplinary process of evaluation, treatment, rehabilitation, functional testing and training in sport-specific skills.

In epicondylitis and epitrochleitis, rest is compulsory for a minimum of 3 weeks and in severe cases, immobilization in a cast is often necessary to fix the elbow at a right angle and the wrist to block prono-supination. Nonsteroidal anti-inflammatory drugs, analgesics and muscle relaxants are always necessary as well as application of ice, physiotherapy and rehabilitation (ultrasound, anti-inflammatory ionisations, deep transvers massage, stretching). Local corticoid infiltrations are often effective when a rapid effect is needed; surgery is only recommended in cases resisting all treatment.

Overuse shoulder injuries are usually treated with ice, rest for 7–10 days, correction of training program and of technical fault, and a rehab program; sometimes a medical intervention with cortisone injections or surgery is required. A basic rehabilitation program includes general aerobic activity, stretching of all muscle groups involved, specific muscles exercises (especially for scapular stabilizers and rotator cuff exercises), ice and anti-inflammatory drugs, laser, ultrasound and massage.

In reference to dorsalgia and interscapular pain, with regard to acute episodes, functional rest associated with cryotherapy is indicated and in the most serious cases the intake of analgesic and anti-inflammatory drugs (NSAIDs). In chronic forms or in the presence of overloads, decontracting massage therapy and physical rehabilitation therapies such as diathermy, high power lasers and ultrasound can be very useful.

1.5 Prevention Strategies

To prevent overuse injuries in archery, shooting technique should be relaxed and efficient and muscle strength should be developed. The drawing force may be a protective factor from injuries. Special attention should be given to a strict linear force transmission from the bow arm to the shoulder girdle, especially when athletes become tired. Effective technique depends on proper balance of strength and flexibility. Warm-up, stretch and strengthening are used in conjunction with proper form to prevent injury. Strengthening the four rotator cuff muscles is essential. Gentle stretching of the rotator cuff muscles can aid in prevention of injuries when done on a regular consistent basis, especially before and after exercise. Not only arm, shoulder and back muscles, but also leg and trunk muscles need to be trained to give the athlete adequate stability. Archery also requires the archer to have a very stable base of support to ensure that the bow and sighting mechanism are held stationary during the shot. This base must be secure in whatever foot position the archer finds themselves. The trasversus abdomens, the deepest of the four abdominal muscles, the multifidus in the back and the internal oblique abdominal are the muscles responsible for low back stability.

However the muscles involved with scapular stabilization, the rhomboids, inferior and middle trapezius, and the pelvic stabilizers must be trained to work as a team. Efficient, timely and strong use of these muscles co-contracting are essential in holding a strong posture against gravity, wind or when standing on uneven surfaces such as those found in field archery. Drawing weight should be chosen according to the archer's constitution (use light bows with young archers). If the archer is working very near their maximum level on a regular basis or during practice, they have no reserve strength left to accommodate adverse weather condition, stress and tension associated with tournament conditions, clicker troubles or shoot off's. The archer must always emphasize the quality of the shot not the quantity of arrows. As a huge number of arrows shot during the training increases precision but also represent a risk of overuse injuries, archers and coaches should focus on perfect technique, especially in beginners. Additional strength training may prevent overuse. Athletes should be aware that asymmetrical loads should be compensated via weight training (both sides must be trained equally to prevent significant muscle imbalance). A complete, well chosen conditioning and training program combines technical practices with general cardio vascular fitness, general shoulder and back strengthening programs, specific rotator cuff and scapular stabilizer strengthening programs, flexibility and muscular endurance.

In order to prevent duration and frequency of painful episodes of dorsalgia, it is necessary to take some precautions, such as avoiding overloads and direct traumas, performing regular postural re-education exercises (core stability) and strengthening the back muscles and maintaining a constant body weight with a percentage of fat mass appropriate for sports activity.

Carefully maintaining sports gear and checking for damage may prevent acute injuries. All competitive archers wear protective gear such as an arm guard and tab anyway, which explains low injury rates in this group of participants.

References

1. Ertan H. Injury patterns among Turkish archers. Shield Res J Phys Educ Sports Sci. 2006;1.
2. Ergen E, Hibner K. Sports medicine and science in archery; 2008.
3. Niestroj K, Küpper T, Schöffl V. Acute and overuse injuries in elite archers. J Sports Med Phys Fitness. 2018;58(7-8):1063–70.
4. Kaur Grover J, Kumar Sinha AG. Prevalence of shoulder pain in competitive archery. Asian J Sports Med. 2017;8(1):e40971.
5. Mann DL, et al. Shoulder injuries in archery. Can J Sport Sci. 1989;14(2):85–92.

Athletics: Jumping

2

Gian Luigi Canata and Valentina Casale

2.1 Characteristics of the Sport

Regular jumping events in Track and Field include high jump, long jump, triple jump, and pole vault.

The goal of jumping is to obtain the longest distance, which may be vertical or horizontal, depending on the discipline. In all cases, however, the horizontal speed reached at the end of the run-up is turned into vertical speed [1].

The Fosbury flop is the most used technique in high jump since 1968, when a college track athlete standardized this new technique twisting the body to leap over the bar faceup and backward. It begins with an approach of several bounding steps toward the bar, in a J-shaped run which starts straight and curves at the end. The straight part of the run-up helps the athlete obtaining speed and momentum, while the curve naturally pulls the jumper's body into a slight turn. The athlete then uses the muscles of legs and buttocks to spring into the air. Head, shoulders, and torso clear the crossbar backward with the chest and belly in a supine position, boosting the waist to pull their hips up and over the crossbar. Once the midsection has cleared the crossbar, the jumper bends at the waist, draws the knees toward the chest to snap the legs and feet up and over the crossbar. The athlete then lands on the shoulders, usually moving into a backward somersault.

The long jump technique has remained basically the same since the beginning of modern athletics. The athlete sprints down a runway, jumps up from a wooden take-off board, flies in the air and lands in a pit of sand. A successful long jump requires high horizontal velocity, muscle power for an effective take-off, and good coordination to perform the take-off, flight, and landing maneuver.

At the take-off moment, the greatest possible vertical speed must be maintained, minimizing any loss of the horizontal speed obtained during the approach run [2]. The greater the runner's velocity at the instant they begin the leap, the greater the body's momentum will be, and the farther they will travel horizontally until gravity pulls them back down. It is well known, in fact, that good long jumpers are good to excellent sprinters, without exception.

In the flight phase, arm swing improves jump height by increasing the height and the velocity of the body's center of gravity at take-off; it contributes to the total body momentum and increases the peak magnitude of the vertical ground reaction force.

G. L. Canata (✉)
Centre of Sports Traumatology, Koelliker Hospital, TORINO, Italy
e-mail: studio@ortosport.it

V. Casale
Centre of Sports Traumatology, Koelliker Hospital, Turin, Italy

© The Author(s), under exclusive license to Springer-Verlag GmbH, DE, part of Springer Nature 2022
G. L. Canata, H. Jones (eds.), *Epidemiology of Injuries in Sports*,
https://doi.org/10.1007/978-3-662-64532-1_2

During landing, the athlete must pass forward the mark made by the feet without sitting back, to avoid the risk of decreasing the distance of the jump.

Triple jump consists of a linear approach run, followed by a hop, a step, and a jump into the sand. The hop begins at the wooden take-off board, then the athlete performs a series of three controlled horizontal jumps before landing in the sand pit. First the jumper must take off on one foot, landing on the same foot; then he takes one long stride, landing on the opposite foot; from that foot the athlete leaps forward, landing into the sand.

A triple jumper, more than the long jumper, combines velocity and momentum with extra motions of the arms, legs, and torso before jumping, helping the center of gravity to move higher. It especially happens during the third and final jump.

The pole vault requires several of the same skills as high jumping, such as the ability to control and maneuver the body around its center of gravity. It consists of seven different phases: the run-up, the plant, the take-off, the swing phase, the rock-back, the inversion position, and the crossbar clearance.

As in the other jump disciplines, the athlete begins with a linear approach run, initially fast but relaxed, then gradually changed to hit top speed just prior to planting the pole. The pole is carried on one side, kept with both hands; during the last steps of the run-up, the jumper raises the hands and pushes forward the pole, until this is planted in the pole vault box.

Now the take-off phase starts: if the athlete carries the pole on the right side of the body, the right arm is extended above the head and close to the pole, while the left arm pushes forward against the pole; the take-off leg is fully extended and close to the pole, while the swing leg is bent at the hip and the knee. During this phase, the pole begins to bend under the effect of the jumper's momentum, storing energy, then both the pole and the athlete rotate using the kinetic energy produced during the run-up and transformed into potential energy. As the pole bends and recoils, the jumper keeps rotating and then pulls up on the pole, reaching the crossbar feet first, in an inverted position.

During the crossbar clearance, the jumper pushes off from the pole with one hand, still rotating the body to face the crossbar with the torso and arching the body to complete the clearance. Finally, the athlete lands on the mat in a supine position.

2.2 Physiological and Biomechanical Demands on Athletes

Considering the long jump as exemplificative of all the jumping disciplines, there are different biomechanical requests according to the several phases of this practice: run-up, take-off, flight, and landing. The objective of each phase is always the same, regardless of the athlete's gender or ability [2].

Because the flight and the landing phases differ among the four main jumping disciplines, only the run-up and the take-off moments will be biomechanically analyzed and described below:

- Performing a fast and accurate run-up is crucial to achieve a good distance. During this phase, after accelerating to near-maximum speed, the athlete lowers the body during the final few steps and brings it into the position for take-off. Finally, they must place the take-off foot accurately on the take-off board.
- It may be assumed that the main cause of variations in jump distance among athletes is probably given by muscular strength.
- Accuracy is also important because the jumper must place the take-off foot close to, but not over, the take-off board. In order to do this, before take-off they must use a visual control strategy during the last few strides to perform some adjustments with the smallest possible loss of horizontal speed [2].
- Furthermore, in the transition from run-up to take-off, the jumper must lower the center of body mass to give a large vertical range of motion over which to generate upward velocity. If correctly performed, this passage allows a minimal downward vertical velocity to the center of body mass at touchdown; conse-

quently, the upward vertical impulse exerted by the jumper during the take-off produces the highest possible vertical velocity.

- In order to take full advantage of the run-up velocity, the take-off technique must be appropriate.

- After placing the take-off foot well ahead of the center of body mass, the jumper's body pivots up and over the take-off foot, while the take-off leg rapidly flexes and extends.

- At the take-off, a "pawing" action is advisable: the take-off leg should be swept down and back toward the athlete. This passage helps to reduce the breaking force experienced by the jumper during the first stages of the take-off.

- These passages basically follow the physics law of "projectile motion," exploiting both the take-off velocity and the take-off angle. The jumper, in fact, plants the foot ahead of the center of body mass to lengthen the duration of the ground contact, hence counteracting the reduction of the vertical impulse generation caused by the take-off moment itself.

- However, this consequential increase in vertical propulsive impulse is combined with an unwanted rise in horizontal breaking impulse. To reduce this ratio, the jumper must apply an optimum leg angle at touchdown, which represents a compromise between vertical propulsive impulse and horizontal braking impulse. In the long jump, this angle is about 60–65° to the horizontal.

- From a biomechanical point of view, it is important to note that the jumper pre-tenses the muscles of the take-off leg just before touchdown. The subsequent flexion of the leg is hence due to the unavoidable force of landing, and limited by the eccentric strength of the athlete's leg muscles. To optimize this balance, the jumper must maximally activate these muscles to pivot up the center of body mass over the foot, producing vertical velocity as a merely mechanical process.

- Over 60% of the jumper's final vertical velocity is achieved by the instant of maximum knee flexion; therefore, the pivot mechanism is the single most important technique contributing to create vertical velocity during the take-off moment [2].

- Greater eccentric muscular leg strength provides the athlete with an effective ability to resist flexion of the take-off leg. Furthermore, fast eccentric actions early in the take-off help the muscles to exert large forces, therefore generating large benefits in vertical velocity.

- During the last half of the take-off, the maximum extension of hip, knee, and ankle is associated with a strong swinging of arms and free leg [2]. As a result, the center of body mass gets higher and farther ahead of the take-off line.

2.3   Epidemiology of Injuries

Both vertical and horizontal jumps are characterized by the production of a maximum force in a short period of time: this event causes maximal muscular contractions, with consequent high stress on several areas, especially along the lower extremities.

Jump practice, in fact, requires good sprinting speed, and the physiological stresses are reflected in the common injuries reported among both jumpers and runners.

Injuries developed in jumping activities are associated with jump-landing movements. A "stiffer" landing technique is a risk factor for developing both overuse injuries and acute traumas for its lesser shock absorbing component [3].

It has been reported that a more flexible jumping pattern, with a large post-touchdown ROM and landing time, may reduce the risk of developing injuries such as patellar tendinopathy. It may be obtained by optimizing kinetic chain function by addressing strength, flexibility and joint function, and changing stiff landing patterns, such as small post-touchdown range of motion (ROM) and short landing time.

Patellofemoral injuries are relatively common, with rates up to 30% of knee injuries seen in sports medicine. In particular, they occur with rates up to 20% among athletes participating in jumping sports: for this reason, patellar tendinopathy is also known as "jumper's knee". It is frequently associated with jumping, cutting, and pivoting activities which eccentrically load the patella: the resulting affections may range from contusion, to tendinopathy, instability and avulsion injuries. Injury rates increase up to 53% when considering chronic anterior knee pain, which is often a significant factor affecting the decision to leave sport.

The main risk factors for developing patellar tendinopathy have been recently reported as: joint flexion angles at touchdown, with a consequent reduction of the available range of motion (ROM); small post-touchdown ROM at the joints; high post-touchdown joint angular velocities.

Landing technique affects the patellar tendon more than the take-off technique does, especially during horizontal landing after a forward acceleration.

Other contributing factors to the development of jumper's knee are related to anatomic and muscular factors, such as overall upper leg strength (especially the vastus medialis oblique, the hamstrings and quadriceps flexibility), leg-length discrepancy, or foot pronation.

Furthermore, because jumper's knee typically develops as an overuse injury, a lack of recovery after intense workouts may contribute to the injury mechanism.

Ankle injuries are another example of injuries that occur during jumping practice. An estimated 20–35% of total time lost to injury in running and jumping sports may be attributed to ankle injuries [3].

They include acute Achilles tendon ruptures, ankle sprains, syndesmotic ankle sprains, metatarsal fractures, and midfoot sprains.

The explosive power needed for the take-off moment, in fact, places considerable strain on structures such as the Achilles tendon, calf muscles, and the patellar tendon.

Most tendon ruptures are caused by a rapid eccentric load applied on a stiff foot, as when performing a sudden jump. Partial tendon ruptures are more frequent than total ruptures because they usually result from repetitive overuse injuries and focal degeneration. Ankle sprains, as well as fifth metatarsal base fractures, usually occur after an inversion of a plantar flexed ankle, as when landing on irregular surfaces. Conversely, an external rotation torque applied to the foot induces syndesmotic ankle sprains.

Sports involving repetitive extension and rotation of the lumbar spine, such as in jumping, increase the risk of injury to the posterior elements of the spine, in particular the spondylolysis. It consists in a pars interarticularis defect of a vertebra, a unilateral or bilateral stress fracture, and it usually begins with insidious onset of extension-related low-back pain; the athlete may develop pain with impact, such as during running and jumping.

It has been reported that repetitive microtrauma, together with insufficiency of the muscle–tendon complex, a reduced maximum strength capacity, and trunk muscle fatigue during dynamic loading may be considered as the major causes of back pain among athletes.

Trunk muscle forces provide stability and may counteract high-impact loading during high-intensity activities. Disciplines such as running, hopping, jumping, and landing enhance the impact forces that need compensation. Trunk strength capacity as well as achieving and maintaining good postural and neuromuscular control play a crucial role in jumping mechanics.

Muscle strains of the posterior aspect of the thigh are common in high-speed running or activities requiring significant ranges of motion.

Healthy and strong muscles may prevent injuries; therefore, their training and management are essential. For example, if the middle gluteal muscles are weak or lack control, there will be a large pelvic drop on the side opposite to the stance leg, with a consequent risk of imbalance-related injuries.

Some patellar tracking problems may be caused by muscular weakness, in particular when considering the vastus medialis oblique. It is the only muscle on the medial side of the patella; therefore, in case of its deficiency, the patella may be pulled laterally, especially during the last 20° of extension of the stance phase.

It has been noted that high-level athletes often diligently train power-generating muscles, for instance, the quadriceps and the gluteals, while neglecting, on the other side, some lower limb muscles such as those crossing the ankle joint in the triple or high jumper. In those cases, prevention is better than cure.

Lower limb stress fractures may affect jumpers, more frequently female athletes, and comprise 5% to 30% of all activity-related injuries of the lower extremities.

Tibial fractures are the most common (24% of all stress fractures). Anatomical abnormalities such as foot hyperpronation or faulty jumping techniques can distribute stress unequally through the feet and legs. In children, tibial stress fractures are commonly observed in the anterior proximal one third of the bone, while in adults, they seem to be highly prevalent in the junction of the middle and distal one thirds. Tension stress is primarily responsible for anterior stress fractures of the tibia and nonunion is more common than anteromedial fractures.

Ten percent of stress fractures occur in the fibula, mainly in the distal one third.

As for the tarsal bones, navicular stress fractures are the most common. They are typically linear and located in the central one third of the bone with a risk of displacement if not diagnosed.

Athletes with a varus foot or knee are more prone to fifth metatarsal fractures.

Risk factors for developing a lower extremity stress fracture, especially a fibular one, include a rapid increase in training programs, female gender, hormonal or menstrual disturbances, low bone turnover rate, decreased thickness of cortical bone, nutritional deficiencies, poor flexibility, inadequate muscle strength, a "type A" behavior pattern (TABP), and much more. Among all these factors, it may be said that stress fractures generally result from a repetitive injury that over time exceeds the intrinsic ability of the bone to repair itself. An aircast splinting is recommended in the case of severe tibial stress fractures, instead of a normal cast for mid-shaft fractures. Intramedullary nailing and/or grafting is advised after six months of no improvement with a conservative approach, or for elite athletes. In case of metatarsal stress fractures, a wood-soled shoe or a casting for four to six weeks is recommended.

Sex differences have been found when analyzing landing movement patterns: male athletes perform risky movements mainly on the sagittal plane (such as landing heel to toe, reduced knee and trunk flexion at initial contact, and limited trunk flexion during landing), while females on the frontal plane (with knee valgus at initial ground contact and maximum knee flexion, or a more frontal plane movement during landing, and more frontal plane errors).

2.4 Rehabilitation and Return to Play

It is important to consider that the human body reacts to high loads differently; thus, athletes of similar level may not tolerate the same training load. Therefore, rehabilitation programs must be adjusted not only according to the site and the degree of injury but also depending on the athlete's individual characteristics and their specific demands.

An essential aspect of the physical training is trunk stabilization, both for recovery and for preventing future injuries. The exercise regimen should stimulate a synergic action of the deep abdominal muscles, especially the internal and transverse oblique muscles, as well as the adductors and the extensors of the lumbar tract.

Core strengthening is fundamental not only for those athletes with low back pain but also for those with lower extremity injuries; reinforcing trunk muscles provides active stiffening and reduces spinal loading, while connecting the upper and lower limbs through the abdominal fascial system.

A further important aspect of a recovery program is to ensure a complete ROM in the joints of the body, in particular those at the lower extremities (hip, knee, and ankle).

The athlete's ability to use the elastic and neural benefits of the stretch–shorten cycle (SSC) together with force and rate of excursion of the activated muscles during a contraction are of paramount importance in a jump performance. Higher forces are associated with a shorter amortisation time from the eccentric to the concentric phase, as well as a greater energy stored in the series elastic component.

A previous muscle contraction may acutely decrease or enhance force production in a subsequent motor activity. Force decline is known as fatigue, while a force increase is called postactivation potentiation (PAP). Consequently, a performance enhancement depends on the prevalence of PAP mechanisms over fatigue mechanisms. For this reason a proper conditioning activity (CA) protocol which may induce PAP is advisable in every sports activity.

The effectiveness of PAP in jumping disciplines is determined by the ability to sprint faster and to jump higher, especially during the run-up and the take-off phases. As in several other sports-performance settings, the most appropriate and effective CA to induce PAP in jumping disciplines is plyometric exercises.

Some authors have recently proposed to perform plyometric exercises during the rest intervals (generally from 7 to 12 min) between jump attempts. During these intervals, the athlete may use a conditioning exercise aiming to improve performance, while wearing appropriate clothing, performing bouts of mild stretching, submaximal jumping, and other exercises separated by short periods of rest.

An example of these suggested series of plyometric exercises consists in three 2-legged rebound vertical jumps, performed 3 min before each attempt: it has been proved that it progressively increases the vertical velocity at the take-off, while it does not influence the horizontal velocity during the run-up phase.

Plyometrics is a form of "ballistic training" developed to improve jump performance capabilities. It has also been reported that it helps strength, running economy, agility, and sprint ability. Furthermore, it may sharpen landing techniques (by reducing valgus stress and strain), increase eccentric muscle control, and enhance knee flexion and hamstrings activity: this last action reduces landing forces and minimizes the risk of non-contact injuries.

2.5 Prevention Strategies

The general risk factors for sports injuries are mentioned below, and approaching those aspects may help in managing and preventing jumping injuries as well [4]:

- Lack of warm-up,
- Inadequate fitness and physical weakness,

- Inappropriate training,
- Lack of recovery,
- Biomechanical imbalances and anatomical factors,
- Inadequate skill/technique,
- Inappropriate footwear or clothing,
- Lack of protective safety equipment,
- Inappropriate environment,
- Prior injury.

An effective prevention program should therefore improve the mental quality of training, paying high attention to the warm-up phase (increasing the body and muscle temperatures, strengthening the elasticity of muscles and the oxygen-transportation capability), and applying active and passive protection measures (such as wearing the right shoes but also reducing training loads in case of fatigue). The correction of technical errors is also mandatory to avoid the risk of further injuries.

Injuries may be predisposed by intrinsic and extrinsic risk factors: from anatomical and biomechanical characteristics (such as *genu valgum*), strength or flexibility imbalances, to abnormal gait biomechanics, or training errors and improper jumping technique.

An important risk factor for developing jump-related injuries is a "stiffer" landing strategy, mainly due to a poor active motion in the lower extremity joints, as well as an increased valgus position of the knee during the landing maneuver. Although stiffness is also age-related, this problem can be solved by landing with greater knee flexion and ankle plantar flexion.

As cited above, female athletes show a greater risk of knee injuries than male jumpers due to a larger Q-angle which causes a valgus stress and weakness in the surrounding muscles. Plyometrics may optimize these attitudes, but plyometric training was historically thought to be unsafe among youth athletes, and a specific level of strength (back squat ≥150% of body mass) was considered as prerequisite.

Nevertheless, young female athletes (aged between 12 and 18 years) with minimal plyometric training experience have recently demonstrated to improve vertical jump and reduce injury risks. This concept has also been confirmed by the emerging youth development research.

Recently, the optimal energy, nutrient and fluid recommendations for athletes has been outlined. They basically suggest that:

- Nutrition programs should be personalized to the athlete, depending on sports discipline, food preferences, and personal responses to other prevention strategies.
- Training and nutrition interact to influence functional and metabolic adaptation capability of the body.

References

1. MacKay J. Up, up, and away: jumping events and the pole vault. In: Track and field - Science behind sports. Farmington Hills: Greenhaven Publishing LLC; 2011. p. 35–47.
2. Linthorne NP. Biomechanics of the long jump. In: Hong Y, Bartlett R, editors. Routledge handbook of biomechanics and human movement science – Routledge international handbooks. Abingdon: Routledge; 2008. p. 340–53.
3. Ortiz C, Wagner E, Fernandez G. Athletic injuries. In: Valderrabano V, Easley M, editors. Foot and ankle sports orthopaedics. Springer; 2017. p. 421–6.
4. Bird S, Brid SR, Black N, et al. An overview of sports injuries: types, causes and prevention. In: Sports injuries: causes, diagnosis, treatment and prevention. Therapy in practice. Cheltenham: Stanley Thornes; 1997. p. 1–9.

Athletics: Long-Distance Running

3

Theodorakys Marín Fermín
and Emmanuel Papakostas

3.1 Long-Distance Running Athlete Definition

Running events ≥3000 m and ≤marathon are considered long-distance races according to the International Association of Athletics Federation (IAAF) [1]. However, the lack of consistency defining a runner and their classification and level has been reported by several authors [2–8]. The estimation of volume and intensity of running should be considered during the design of investigations to allow classifying the data according to the runner's level [2].

Due to the available epidemiologic studies from marathon races, reporting injury epidemiology separately from other long-distance racing events has become a tendency [9]. However, for this chapter, athletes participating in the mentioned events will be addressed as long-distance runners.

3.2 Incidence and Prevalence

Analysis of existing evidence regarding incidence and prevalence constitutes a challenge for any researcher. Heterogeneity in injury definition and time exposure bias statistical analysis, potentially considering symptomatic functional athletes as injured while performing [2].

The vast majority of the literature has been obtained during competition events. While these studies may offer essential information, they are not representative for the entire season and are not enough to understand risk and injury during longer periods and across athletes from different competitive levels [9, 10]. The consensus statement developed by Timpka et al. (2014) aims to standardize data collection [10]. Improvements in the quality of the obtained data will enhance our understanding of long-distance runners' injuries.

According to Edouard et al. (2019), long-distance running athlete's injuries account for 11.9% (10.6% in men and 14.1% in women, respectively) and marathon athlete's injuries for 9.2% of injuries during 2007–2018 International Championship events [9].

A systematic review of 17 studies conducted by van Gent et al. (2007) reported a range of lower limb injuries incidence between 19.4% and 79.3% in long-distance runners. The incidence raised to 92.4% when non-lower limb injuries were also considered [11, 12].

T. Marín · E. Papakostas (✉)
ASPETAR, Orthopaedic and Sports Medicine
Hospital, Doha, Qatar
e-mail: emmanouil.papakostas@aspetar.com;
papacostas@the-mis.gr

© The Author(s), under exclusive license to Springer-Verlag GmbH, DE, part of Springer Nature 2022
G. L. Canata, H. Jones (eds.), *Epidemiology of Injuries in Sports*,
https://doi.org/10.1007/978-3-662-64532-1_3

Long-distance running events, marathons, and combined events present the highest number of injuries per 1000 registered athletes and per 1000 athlete days [9] Incidences reported range from 2.5 to 33 injuries depending on the population and follow-up, and 89.4 in marathon running per 1000 h of running [7, 13–16].

van Poppel et al.'s (2016) meta-analysis revealed a weighted injury incidence of 17.8 and 7.7 in novice runners and recreational runners (95% CI), respectively [12]. For those training for marathons, the yearly incidence rate can be higher and has been reported to be as high as 90%, according to Satterthwaite et al. (1993) [17–19].

On the subject of prevalence, injuries have been reported in 54.8% of runners [11, 12, 20, 21]. Chang et al.'s (2011) cross-sectional study estimated that at least one-third of the recreational runners experience a minimum of one injury per season, 44.4% of participants reported having previous injuries in the lower limb and 16.1% had multiple injuries by the time of competition [20].

3.3   Risk Factors

While running is commonly accepted as a healthy habit and fitness improving exercise, long-distance running increases demands on the musculoskeletal system and subsequently the risk of injury. Recreational runners have several times greater incidence of injuries compared to their peers playing football or handball [14].

Systematic reviews and meta-analysis by van Gent et al. (2007), Videbaek et al. (2015), and Hulme et al. (2016) have provided useful information about risk factors and determinants for injuries in long-distance running [7, 11, 16].

There is limited evidence for risk of injury in systemic and health factors such as increased age and sex. Nevertheless, Fields (2011) has alerted about the increasing enrollment of ≥40 years old runners in long-distance events, representing a third of the participants. Thus, different patterns of injuries are expected in this age group [22]. Lower leg length difference, greater left tubercle-sulcus angle, greater knee varus, greater height in

male runners, drinking alcohol, participation in cycling and aerobics, and positive medical history are also reported [11].

Concerning training/running factors, limited evidence shows increased risk in greater training frequency in male runners, running the whole year through, greater training distance in female runners, participation in races of greater distance, women running on concrete surfaces, competitive male runners, increase in days of training per week, increase in training distance per week, level of experience in running, use of more shoes for running, and shoe age [11, 17].

Controversy in weight and body mass index compels a thorough approach depending on the level of the athlete and training workload [11].

Concerning runner experience, more experienced runners seem to be at less risk. A timeframe of 5 years has been found to lessen the injury risk significantly, and novice runners are at greater risk than recreational ones [7, 8, 11, 12, 14, 17, 18]. Vitez et al.'s (2017) findings suggest male gender, 1–3 years of running history, and a history of previous injuries as risk factors for lifetime running injury [21].

3.4   Injury Characteristics: Location, Etiology, and Type

Long-distance running injuries predominantly affect the lower limbs. The knee is the most common location of injuries (7.2–50%) [8, 11, 20, 21] followed by lower leg (including Achilles tendon) (9–32.2%), foot (5.7–39.3%) [8, 11, 20, 21], and thigh (3.4–38.1%) [8, 11].

Edouard et al. (2019) reported injuries in lower leg (36.9–40.8%), skin (42.9–48%), and muscles (24.5–29.8) with similar incidence in both genders. No significant gender differences in injury characteristics between long-distance and marathon runners were found. Traumatic injuries represented almost half of the injuries in long-distance races, while overuse injuries were encountered in 69.1–69.8% of marathon runners [9].

In contrast to short distance runners affected mostly by thigh injuries, long-distance athletes are prone to injure their lower leg [9].

3.5 Injury Time Loss

Time-loss data is scarce. It can be obtained from studies with time-loss injury definition and competition surveys; therefore, careful interpretation should be considered [7].

A marathon study by Holmich et al. (1988) revealed that 43% of elite marathon runners suffered injuries severe enough to prevent them from training [23]. A significantly higher incidence of time-loss injuries during competition has been reported compared to those sustained during training [24].

Vitez et al. (2017) surveyed time-loss injuries from almost 20,000 marathon runners. While 65% did not experience running-related injuries, 19% of the participants reported minor problems that required a maximum absence of 2 weeks, 10% moderate with 3–4 weeks, and 7% injuries that kept them out of track for more than 4 weeks [21].

Edouard et al. (2019) revealed no time-loss (36–49.0%) or time loss of up to 7 days (25.5–30.2%) in male long-distance runners and marathon runners, respectively. In contrast, no time loss (39.3–40%) or time loss of up to 7 days (27.3–29.8%) were found in their female counterparts [9]. The presence of 8–28 days of time loss (23.8%) was observed in female long-distance runners, suggesting the incidence of more severe injuries in this group [9].

3.6 Specific Injuries

In the available evidence for the incidence of injuries in long-distance runners, specific injuries are not stated, except for Achilles tendinopathies [5]. There is limited information and a severe lack when comparing different level athletes. However, based on our experience, a selection of specific injuries discussion will contribute to an understanding concerning complaints of these athletes.

Achilles tendinopathies may represent the most frequent tendinopathy among runners and is a common cause of disability [4, 25, 26]. The increasing participation of athletes in long-distance races has raised its incidence in the past decades, reaching 9.1–10.9%, and prevalence 6.2–9.5% [4,

25, 26]. In elite-level runners, the lifetime incidence is estimated between 7% and 9% [25].

Risk factors such as increased age and force distribution in running patterns have limited evidence for mid-portion Achilles tendinopathy, but having a previous Achilles tendon disorder is probably the most important factor to consider [27]. Also, gastrocnemius and soleus muscle overloading and running on the sand surface are potential causes of Achilles tendinopathies [28–30].

Iliotibial band syndrome has been identified as the most common cause of lateral knee pain in running athletes [31, 32]. Incidence has been reported in 16% of runners [33]. While no gender association has been found, prevalence seems to be higher in female runners (9.8% vs. 6.8%) and may have the same behavior when considering lifetime prevalence [33, 34]. The evidence correlating knee or foot alignment and leg length with iliotibial band syndrome is inconclusive [33].

Stress fractures of the tibia, ankle, and foot are considered a major cause of disability in athletes of all kinds and levels. Although the incidence is less than 1% among the athletic population in general, it can be as high as 15% in runners. Available data is scarce for a correct epidemiologic assessment of these injuries, as the source of most of the studies come from the military and college/high-school population, but a higher risk in the female is shown [35–39]. To analyze the population at risk, we consider appropriately extrapolating data on medial tibial stress syndrome, which has an incidence range from 8% to 20.0% and a 9.5% prevalence [2, 4].

Specific incidences have been reported for metatarsals 20% [40–42], navicular 15–32% [41, 43], fibula 6.6% [40], and medial malleolus 0.6–4.1% [41, 42]. Disturbances in menstruation and low bone mineral density are potentially associated with a significantly increased risk of stress fracture development [16, 39].

3.7 Prevention

Eduard et al. (2019) suggest focused attention on screening athletes participating in long-distance races during the season and 1 month before the event interviewing dietary and menstrual history in the female athlete [9, 39]. Overuse injuries and under conditioning seems to have a narrow gap; thus, workload and recovery/adaptation should be the target when considering the design of prevention programs for long-distance running athletes [11].

Advising athletes to run a maximum of 64 km/week, adopting interval training, and increasing training distances every week (for injury knee prevention) may result in a successful preventive intervention [8, 11, 12].

References

1. International Association of Athletics Federations (IAAF). 2019. https://www.worldathletics.org/
2. Francis P, Whatman C, Sheerin K, Hume P, Johnson MI. The proportion of lower limb running injuries by gender, anatomical location, and specific pathology: a systematic review. J Sports Sci Med. 2019;18(1):21–31.
3. Kluitenberg B, van Middelkoop M, Diercks R, van der Worp H. What are the differences in injury proportions between different populations of runners? A systematic review and meta-analysis. Sports Med. 2015;45(8):1143–61.
4. Lopes A, Hespanhol L, Yeung S, Costa L. What are the main running-related musculoskeletal injuries? A systematic review. Sports Med. 2012;42(10):891–905.
5. van der Worp M, de Wijer A, van Cingel R, Verbeek A, Nijhuisvan der Sanden M, Staal J. The 5- or 10-km Marikenloop Run: a prospective study of the etiology of running-related injuries in women. J Orthop Sports Phys Ther. 2016;46(6):462–70.
6. Nielsen R, Buist I, Sorensen H, Lind M, Rasmussen S. Training errors and running related injuries: a systematic review. Int J Sports Phys Ther. 2012;7(1):58–75.
7. Videbaek S, Bueno A, Nielsen R, Rasmussen S. Incidence of running-related injuries per 1000 h of running in different types of runners: a systematic review and meta-analysis. Sports Med. 2015;45(7):1017–26.
8. van Middelkoop M, Kolkman J, Van Ochten J, Bierma-Zeinstra S, Koes B. Prevalence and incidence of lower extremity injuries in male marathon runners. Scand J Med Sci Sports. 2008;18:140–4.
9. Edouard P, Navarro L, Branco P, Gremeaux V, Timpka T, Junge A. Injury frequency and characteristics (location, type, cause, and severity) differed significantly among athletics ('track and field') disciplines during 14 international championships (2007–2018): implications for medical service planning. Br J Sports Med. 2019; pii: bjsports-2019-100717
10. Timpka T, Alonso J, Jacobsson J, et al. Injury and illness definitions and data collection procedures for use in epidemiological studies in athletics (track and field): consensus statement. Br J Sports Med. 2014;48(7):483–90.
11. van Gent R, Siem D, van Middelkoop M, van Os A, Bierma-Zeinstra S, Koes B. Incidence and determinants of lower extremity running injuries in long-distance runners: a systematic review. Br J Sports Med. 2007;41:469–80.
12. van Poppel D, de Koning J, Verhagen A, Scholten-Peeters G. Risk factors for lower extremity injuries among half marathon and marathon runners of the Lage Landen Marathon Eindhoven 2012: a prospective cohort study in the Netherlands. Scand J Med Sci Sports. 2016;26(2):226–34.
13. Jakobsen B, Kroner K, Schmidt S, Kjeldsen A. Prevention of injuries in long-distance runners. Knee Surg Sports Traumatol Arthrosc. 1994;2(4):245–9.
14. Jakobsen B, Kroner K, Schmidt S, Jensen J. The frequency of injuries in recreational running races. Ugeskr Laeger. 1988;150(48):2954–6.
15. Lysholm J, Wiklander J. Injuries in runners. Am J Sports Med. 1987;15(2):168–71.
16. Hulme A, Thompson J, Nielsen R, Read G, Salmon P. Towards a complex system approach in sports injury research: simulating running-related injury development with agent-based modelling. Br J Sports Med. 2019;53(9):560–9.
17. Fredericson M, Misra A. Epidemiology and aetiology of marathon running injuries. Sports Med. 2007;37(4-5):437–9.
18. Satterthwaite P, Larmer P, Gardiner J, et al. Incidence of injuries and other health problems in the Auckland Citibank Marathon, 1993. Br J Sports Med. 1996;30:324–6.
19. van Mechelen M. Running injuries: a review of the epidemiological literature. Sports Med. 1992;14(5):320–35.
20. Chang W, Shih Y, Chen W. Running injuries and associated factors in participants of ING Taipei Marathon. Phys Ther Sport. 2012;13(3):170–4.
21. Vitez L, Zupet P, Zadnik V, Drobnic M. Running injuries in the participants of Ljubljana Marathon. Zdr Varst. 2017;56(4):196–202.
22. Fields K. Running injuries - changing trends and demographics. Curr Sports Med Rep. 2011;10(5):299–303.
23. Holmich P, Darre E, Jahnsen F, Hartvig-Jensen T. The elite marathon runner: problems during and after competition. Br J Sports Med. 1988;22(1):19–21.
24. Feddermann-Demont N, Junge A, Edouard P, Branco P, Alonso J. Injuries in 13 international athletics championships between 2007–2012. Br J Sports Med. 2014;48(7):513–22.
25. Longo U, Ronga M, Maffulli N. Achilles tendinopathy. Sports Med Arthrosc Rev. 2009;17(2):112–26.
26. Hespanhol L, Carvalho A, Costa L, Lopes A. The prevalence of musculoskeletal injuries in runners: a systematic review. Br J Sports Med. 2011;45:351–2.

27. Knobloch K, Yoon U, Vogt P. Acute and overuse injuries correlated to hours of training in master running athletes. Foot Ankle Int. 2008;29(7):671–6.

28. Nielsen R, Buist I, Sorensen H, et al. Training errors and running related injuries: a systematic review. Int J Sports Phys Ther. 2012;7(1):58–75.

29. Arndt A, Komi P, Bruggemann G, et al. Individual muscle contributions to the in vivo Achilles tendon force. Clin Biomech (Bristol, Avon). 1998;13(7):532–41.

30. Baker RL, Fredericson M. Iliotibial band syndrome in runners: biomechanical implications and exercise interventions. Phys Med Rehabil Clin N Am. 2016;27(1):53–77.

31. Noehren B, Davis I, Hamill J. ASB clinical biomechanics award winner 2006 prospective study of the biomechanical factors associated with iliotibial band syndrome. Clin Biomech (Bristol, Avon). 2007;9:951–6.

32. Fredericson M, Wolf C. Iliotibial band syndrome in runners: innovations in treatment. Sports Med. 2005;35:451–9.

33. Taunton J, Ryan M, Clement D, et al. A retrospective case-control analysis of 2002 running injuries. Br J Sports Med. 2002;2:95–101.

34. Tenforde AS, Sayres LC, McCurdy ML, et al. Overuse injuries in high school runners: lifetime prevalence and prevention strategies. PM R. 2011;2:125–31.

35. Hulkko A, Orava S. Stress fractures in athletes. Int J Sports Med. 1987;8(3):221–6.

36. Wentz L, Liu P, Haymes E, et al. Females have a greater incidence of stress fractures than males in both military and athletic populations: a systemic review. Mil Med. 2011;176(4):420–30.

37. Hame S, LaFemina J, McAllister D, et al. Fractures in the collegiate athlete. Am J Sports Med. 2004;32(2):446–51.

38. Changstrom B, Brou L, Khodaee M, et al. Epidemiology of stress fracture injuries among US high school athletes, 2005-2006 through 2012-2013. Am J Sports Med. 2015;43(1):26–33.

39. Greaser M. Foot and ankle stress fractures in the athlete. Orthop Clin North Am. 2016;47(4):809–22.

40. Matheson G, Clement D, McKenzie D, et al. Stress fractures in athletes. A study of 320 cases. Am J Sports Med. 1987;15(1):46–58.

41. Brukner P, Bradshaw C, Khan K, et al. Stress fractures: a review of 180 cases. Clin J Sport Med. 1996;6(2):85–9.

42. Iwamoto J, Takeda T. Stress fractures in athletes: review of 196 cases. J Orthop Sci. 2003;8(3):273–8.

43. Bennell KL, Malcolm SA, Thomas SA, et al. The incidence and distribution of stress fractures in competitive track and field athletes. A twelve-month prospective study. Am J Sports Med. 1996;24(2):211–7.

Athletics: Sprinting

4

Pascal Edouard

4.1 Introduction

Athletics is an Olympic sport composed of several different disciplines, including the sprints (https://www.iaaf.org/disciplines/sprints/100-metres), which consists in running as fast as possible a predetermined distance up to 400 m. The practice of sprints can lead to injuries. Injuries can affect all tissues constituting the musculoskeletal structure (especially muscle and tendon, but also bone, cartilage, ligament or soft tissue), with a sudden or gradual mode of onset, by acute trauma or repeated micro-trauma ('overuse'). These injuries can have an impact not only in sport, with the consequences that this represents in high-level athletes, but also in everyday life (school, work, daily file activities, etc.). Consequently, an optimal management of these injuries, with primary and secondary prevention perspectives, represents an important challenge for all stakeholders involved in athletes.

4.2 Characteristics of Sprints

Initially, as part of the Ancient Olympics, sprints were represented by the 'stade' (192 m race). In more modern times, the 100 yards (91.44 m) was adopted as the foremost sprint. The classic 100 m distance has been part of the Olympics since 1896.

The discipline of sprints includes distances from 100 m to 400 m for outdoor competitions on a 400-m track, and for indoor competitions, distances from 50 m and 60 m on a home straight track and from 200 m to 400 m on a 200-m track. For all races, athletes start from blocks, and run in separated lanes (except for the relay 4 × 400 m during which athletes are all together after 500 m of the race). For the 50 m, 60 m, and 100 m, athletes race down the home straight. For 200 m and 400 m, athletes run 100 m around a bend and 100 m down the home straight (until reaching the predetermined distance).

The performance of the athlete is the time measured between the start of the race (given by the shot of the starter) and when they cross the finish line, and the ranking position of the order of arrival of the athletes. A reaction time (measured by sensors in the starting pistol and on the

P. Edouard (✉)
Inter-University Laboratory of Human Movement Science (LIBM EA 7424), University of Lyon, University Jean Monnet, Saint-Etienne, France

Sports Medicine Unit, Faculty of Medicine, Department of Clinical and Exercise Physiology, University Hospital of Saint-Etienne, Saint-Etienne, France

European Athletics Medical and Anti Doping Commission, European Athletics Association (EAA), Lausanne, Switzerland
e-mail: pascal.edouard@univ-st-etienne.fr

blocks) of less than 0.1 s is deemed a false start, athletes are thus recalled, and the responsible athlete of the false start is disqualified.

4.3 Physiological and Biomechanical Demands of Sprints

Understanding the physiological and biomechanical demands of sprints is not only of great interest because of their critical value to performance but also for injury management and prevention. Indeed, better understanding the body's requirements/constraints to be performant can help to appropriately prepare athletes in order to overcome the constraints of the sport, to thus limit the occurrence of an injury, and after an injury to limit the risk of recurrence.

Sprints have been divided into four phases: start from the blocks, acceleration, constant velocity and deceleration of the velocity [1]. The start is an important component of a sprint because, although sprinters typically spend less than 0.4 s pushing against the blocks, they exit the blocks with velocities already around 30% of their maximum. Neural-motor integration is clearly one aspect that is important in this acceleration phase, as sprinters must sense and respond to the starting signal as rapidly as possible. During the acceleration phase, the athlete's aim is to produce great force/power and generate high velocity [1]. Forward orientation of ground reaction force has been shown to be a stronger determinant of field sprint performance than the overall magnitude of vertical or resultant ground force reaction, and hip extensor muscles (*gluteus maximus* and hamstring muscles) playing a key role in this horizontal force production [2]. During the constant-speed phase, the events immediately before and during the braking phase are important in increasing power and efficiency of movement in the propulsion phase [1]. Regarding the deceleration phase, the aim is to limit the decrease of velocity by continuing as long as possible to produce forward oriented force or limit its decrease [1].

Sprints are short duration events, from approximately 6 s–60 s, requiring energy from anaerobic alactic and lactic metabolisms. For short sprints (duration <10 s), energy rely predominantly on the ATP-PCr system to supply the ATP needed for muscle contraction, whereas anaerobic glycolysis provides a greater percentage of the required ATP as distance increases. Determinants of the performance come more from mechanical aspects (i.e. neuro-muscular and technical aspects) than metabolic one. These mechanical aspects include (but are not limited to): leg strength, power and stiffness, and muscle mass, fibre type composition and fascicle length (e.g. large cross-sectional area of type II fibres in the leg muscles) [1].

4.4 Epidemiology of Injuries in Sprints

As in many sports, the practice of sprints can lead to a risk of injuries, which can affect all tissues constituting the musculoskeletal structure (especially muscle and tendon, but also bone, cartilage, ligament or soft tissue) [3, 4]. A good view of the extent of the problem is a fundamental first step in injury prevention [3].

4.4.1 Injuries in Sprints During the Entire Athletics Season

There are few studies detailing the epidemiology of athletics injuries during the entire athletics season, and this is also true for sprints.

In 1994, D'Souza [5] reported in a retrospective cohort study of all-level athletes that 67.5% of sprinters sustained at least one injury during one athletics season. The most frequent locations were back (29.6%), foot (22.2%), hamstring (18.5%) and shin (18.5%).

In 1996, Bennell and Crossley [6] reported in a retrospective cohort study of all-level athletes that the most frequent diagnoses in sprinters were hamstring strain (38%), stress fracture (17%) and knee overuse (14%).

In 2013, Jacobsson et al. [7] reported in a prospective cohort study of high-level athletes that 65% of sprinters sustained at least one injury during one athletics season. All injuries were reported as non-traumatic injuries. The most frequent locations were hip/groin/thigh (37.5%) and Achilles tendon/ankle/foot/toe (37.5%). The most frequent diagnosis in sprinters was hamstring strain (23.5%).

4.4.2 Injuries in Sprints During Major International Championships

During 14 international athletics championships from 2007 to 2018, a total of 382 injuries were collected by the national medical teams (physicians and/or physiotherapists) and/or by the local organising committee physicians among the 4449 athletes registered in sprints [4]. This represented 25% of all injuries recorded during these 14 championships, making the sprints the discipline with the highest number/proportion of injuries [4]. This corresponded to 86 injuries per 1000 registered: 95 injuries per 1000 registered male sprinters and 75 injuries per 1000 female sprinters, with significantly more injuries in male than female sprinters (relative risk of 1.27 (95% confidence interval 1.04–1.54)) [4].

Regarding the characteristics of the injuries, most injuries of male sprinters were located at the thigh (52%), affected the muscles (68%), were caused by overuse (43%) or trauma (39%), and were expected to lead to no time-loss (39%), time-loss of up to 7 days (24%) or 8 to 28 days (23%) [4]. For female sprinters, most injuries were located at the thigh (38%), the foot (13%) or the trunk (12%), affected muscles (49%) or skin (15%), were caused by overuse (51%), and were expected to lead to no time-loss (50%) or time-loss of up to 7 days (23%) [4]. There were some differences between male and female sprinters for the distribution of injury location and injury type, but not with regard to injury cause or severity [4]. There were no significant differences in injury characteristics between outdoor and indoor championships [4].

4.4.3 Summary of the Epidemiology of Injuries in Sprints

As an overall picture of the injuries sustained by sprinters, typical injuries are hamstring muscle injuries, Achilles tendinopathies, stress fractures and low back pain.

4.5 Specific Injuries of Sprinters

4.5.1 Hamstring Muscle Injuries in Sprinters

By far, the most common injury in sprints is the hamstring muscle injury. This represented approximately 50% of all injuries in sprinters during international athletics championships, leading to an estimated mean time loss of 11 days (with a standard deviation of 10 days) [8]. During the season, according to the study from Jacobsson et al. [7], hamstring muscle injuries were a quarter of all injuries sustained by athletes during one season. Askling et al. [9] reported time to return to sports after a hamstring muscle injury in sprinters from 20 to 140 days, highlighting the impact of this injury for sprinters.

Some factors have been reported to be associated with hamstring injuries in sprints in athletics: sex (male athletes), age (older athletes) and hamstring-to-quadriceps imbalance (the isokinetic hamstring/quadriceps ratio less than 60% at 180°/s).

Hamstring muscle injury is characterized by more or less acute pain in the posterior thigh compartment with a functional impact ranging from simple discomfort to total functional impotence. The diagnosis is essentially clinical. The interview will have a prominent place and the physical examination will confirm the hypotheses and refine the diagnosis. The interview will search to determine the mechanisms and mode of onset of the pain/injury, and then the repercussion for the athletes. The clinical examination will analyse the repercussion through the palpation, range of motion and strength testing. Paraclinical examinations can be performed to eliminate a differential diagnosis or even specify the diagnosis.

From the first moments after injury and during the first days, it is currently advisable to be careful not to aggravate the injury. The protocol POLICE: Protection, Optimal Loading, Ice, Compression and Elevation, and now extended to the PEACE and LOVE protocol [10] is followed (even if it still lacks solid scientific evidence). Walking or even certain physical activities may be allowed if they do not create any pain and do not lead to aggravation of the lesion and oedema. The rehabilitation should start early, in order to favour muscle tissue healing, and by respecting the rule of no pain in order to avoid aggravation or recurrence. A global rehabilitation program of progressive increase of the constraints/stresses, based on individual and objective criteria, with a multifactorial approach including a care of all the elements of the propulsion chain of the lower limbs (foot, ankle, leg, knee, thigh, pelvis, trunk) has shown its effectiveness in reducing recurrence compared to conventional rehabilitation approaches only focused on the hamstring muscles [11]. The rehabilitation should also include running exercises and drills, and should be oriented to prepare athletes to sprint.

Return to sports should be progressive, following the return to sport continuum, by progressively increasing the volume and intensity of the physical activities, without any pain, and without any big increase in the intensity. The authorization to return to competition should thus be the logical consequence of the progressive return to sports. An objective evaluation by a health professional is recommended to guide this gradual step by step return to sport. The decision to return the sport is a shared decision, fully involving the athlete, whose health must be at the centre of attention, benefiting from the integrity and caring participation of all stakeholders around the athletes, and taking into account aspects related to the injury and its healing, and the specific characteristics of the sport and its context.

4.5.2 Achilles Tendinopathy in Sprinters

The Achilles tendinopathy is a common injury in athletes practicing sprints (but mainly jumps). During running and jumping activities, the Achilles tendon is undergoing forces ranging from 6 to 14 times bodyweight. Although repetitive tendon loading is an important factor in the development of tendon pathology, it is unclear whether it is entirely responsible for tendon pain because metabolic, genetic, biomechanical factors could also play a role. This is an overuse

injury, but the mode of onset could be gradual or acute. Achilles tendinopathy is often characterized by a history of an insidious onset of pain, often associated with a change in activity such as increased frequency, duration or intensity. Less frequently, pain is reported acutely after a specific incident. At the initial stages, Achilles tendinopathy is typically associated with pain or discomfort at the start of exercises, and pain decreases/disappears with continued activity. With progression of the pathology, pain is felt during exercise and can eventually lead to a cessation of activity. The presence of morning discomfort or pain (often reported as 'stiffness' by the patient) is also frequently associated. The severity of these morning symptoms can be used to indicate the tendons' response to treatment or physical activity.

The interview, physical examination and imaging aim to determine the exact location of the injury (body of the tendon, peri-tendon, bursa, enthesis) and if there is inflammation or not. According to this later point, the treatment will be adapted. If there is inflammation, the treatment will start by trying to limit the chronicization of the inflammation, by activity adaptation (i.e. decreasing load, rest or immobilization), physiotherapy and pharmaceuticals if needed. Then, as for injury without inflammation, the treatment will aim to restore a functional tendon through a number of inter-related components: managing tendon pain with the modification of tendon load and exercise-based rehabilitation programme and adapting the tendon to increasing load. Limiting tendon load is an effective method of decreasing the patient's symptoms to manageable levels and is a crucial part of the rehabilitation programme. Once the patient's symptoms have stabilized, it is important to increase tendon load without increasing symptoms, through a gradual and organized way by initially progressing through the different stages of the rehabilitation programme and gradually adding training and competition loads. Exercises should simulate the individual's maximal sporting function by activating the appropriate muscular activity at suitable loads, speeds and angles. This functional retraining will ensure that the tendon can manage the level of loading required to return to pre-injury levels of activity.

4.5.3 Stress Fractures in Sprinters

Although sprints are explosive disciplines, stress fractures do also exist as one of the frequent diagnosis. They are most frequently located on the foot (navicular tarsal, metatarsal or talus bones), representing high-risk stress fractures. The distinction between low-risk and high-risk types will guide the treatment. A low-risk stress fracture may result in deconditioning and unnecessary time away from activity or sport, and undertreatment of a high-risk fracture can lead to complete fracture or non-union. High-risk stress fractures tend to be subject to tensile force, resulting in a lack of intrinsic stability and eventual formation of a fracture gap, owing to the cortical bone's low resistance to tensile loading. These high-risk stress fractures can be challenging to treat and may require restricted weight-bearing or possibly surgery, in addition to activity modification and/or rest.

The diagnosis should be evoked as soon as the athlete complains about pain in the bone area. The mode of onset could be gradual, with pain occurring during less and less important efforts, but also acute during one specific incident. The most important point to make the diagnosis is to think about this potential injury. The interview will collect arguments in favour of the diagnosis regarding the pain, and the associated factors to stress fractures (e.g. important workload and/or changes in workload, including training, professional activity and daily life). Examination will search to highlight the pain next to the bone, through palpation, percussion and mechanical constraints. Then, the diagnosis will be confirmed by imaging: X-ray, magnetic resonance imaging and/or CT-scan to allow the best characterization of the stress fracture (especially if surgery is discussed). The aim is also to eliminate a differential diagnosis (e.g. osteoid osteoma, chronic osteomyelitis or bone tumour).

The initial treatment is activity restriction, and possibly immobilization. Rest could be asked to overcome the general fatigue context which favours the stress fracture. Surgical treatment is offered to patients with displaced stress fractures, nondisplaced stress fractures with sclerotic margins, patients who fail conservative treatment or patients who cannot tolerate a long period of conservative treatment. A global care is needed to secure all factors favouring the stress fracture.

Return to sports is allowed once tenderness has resolved. Modification of activity may be necessary, such as optimization of training techniques and footwear.

4.5.4 Low Back Pain in Sprinters

Low back pain has also been reported as a common pathology in sprinters. This could be a consequence of the lower leg strengthening programmes (e.g. squats) performed by athletes to increase their strength/power, but also as consequence of the thigh muscles adaptation to training (stiffness of the quadriceps and hamstring muscles leading to change in the pelvic tilt and lumbar curve).

Through interview, physical examination and imaging, a clear diagnosis should be done, in order to propose the most appropriate management. Low back pain can be a consequence of discopathy, isthmic lysis or muscle spasms. All these specific diagnoses should benefit from a specific treatment. In general, these treatments will aim to avoid the pain, restore the motion and function, prepare the athlete for sports, and limit the risk of recurrence. According to the diagnosis, treatment will include a lumbar belt or a stiff corset, adaptation of activities (from rest to decreasing activities), stretching and strengthening, and progressive return to activities.

4.6 Prevention Strategies

The prevention of sprinting-related injuries represents an important challenge for the athletes and all stakeholders around them. Currently and to the best of our knowledge, there is no scientific evidence proven by randomized controlled trials or other high-quality studies on the efficacy of injury prevention measures in athletics, especially in sprinters. However, using an evidence-based approach combining evidence from other sports and experience in athletics, some proposals of injury prevention measures could be done [3, 12].

The preventative approach should be global, multimodal and multifactorial.

As for the general injury and illness prevention at major athletics championships, the 10 tips 'PREVATHLES' could be relevant [12]: (1) Prepare for travel (medical checking, vaccine, time-zone, jet lag, culture, food habits…), (2) Respect athlete characteristics and discipline specificity (sex, endurance/explosive), (3) Educate athletes and their entourages regarding prevention, (4) Vigilance of painful symptoms and subclinical illness markers, (5) Avoid infection risk (washing hands, safe food and drink, avoid contact with sick people, etc.), (6) Train appropriately and optimally (physical conditioning, technical training, load management, psychological preparation), (7) Health status (history of previous injuries, well-being in the month before championships), (8) Lifestyle (good sleep, regular hydration and nutrition with safe water/food, regular fruits and vegetables, improve recovery strategies, etc.), (9) Environmental considerations (heat, cold, air cleaning, changes or climatic conditions), (10) Safety (equipment, rules, own-practice in athletics and extra-sport activities) [12].

In addition, specific tips focused on sprinters could be done through the acronym 'SPRINT':

– Sprint: prepare/train the athlete to run/sprint at maximal velocity, through a progressive approach, including drills and technical skills, and regular exposure to maximal sprints [13];
– Plurifactorial and plurimodal approach, including physical psychological and sociological approaches, and with education of the athletes and stakeholders around them;
– Repair/rehabilitate all injuries until the return to sport and their maximal capabilities;
– Increase capacities of tissues by strengthening, stretching and sensorimotor control training;

– Not neglect pain, and take care of it properly;
– Train appropriately, adapt the load, increase progressively volume and intensity.

Because 'the function creates the organ,' we think that maximal sprinting can help to improve the body capabilities, especially the lower limb, in this sprinting-specific action, for both performance and injury prevention, by being more efficient in sprinting but also to resist the potential damage caused by the sprinting activity [13]. Therefore, we think that maximal sprinting should be considered not only as a part of the problem but also, and more importantly, as a part of the solution [13]. We think that sprint-oriented injury prevention strategies can decrease injuries while also playing a 'win–win' role in improving sprint performance, and could have a higher impact on athletes and coaches' agreement in the approach [13].

References

1. Mero AA, Gregor R. Biomechanics of sprint running. Sports Med. 1992;13(6):376–92.
2. Morin J-B, Gimenez P, Edouard P et al. Sprint acceleration mechanics: the major role of hamstrings in horizontal force production. Front Physiol 2015;6:404.
3. Edouard P, Alonso JM, Jacobsson J et al. Injury prevention in athletics: the race has started and we are on track! New Stud Athl 2015;30(3):69–78.
4. Edouard P, Navarro L, Branco P, Gremeaux V, Timpka T, Junge A. Injury frequency and characteristics differed significantly between athletics disciplines during international championships with meaningful implications for medical service planning. Br J Sports Med. 2019; In press
5. D'SOUZA, D. (1994). Track and field athletics injuries--a one-year survey. Br J Sports Med, 28 (3): 197-202.
6. Bennell KL, Crossley K. Musculoskel- etal injuries in track and field: incidence, distribution and risk factors. Aust J Sci Med Sport. 1996;28(3):69–75.
7. Jacobsson J, Timpka T, Kowalski J, Nilsson S, Ekberg J, Dahlström O, Renström P. Injury patterns in Swedish elite athletics: annual incidence, injury types and risk factors. Br J Sports Med. 2013;47:941–52.
8. Edouard P, Branco P, Alonso JM. Muscle injury is the principal injury type and hamstring muscle injury is the first injury diagnosis during top-level international athletics championships between 2007 and 2015. Br J Sports Med. 2016;50(10):619–30.
9. Askling CM, Tengvar M, Tarassova O, Thorstensson A. Acute hamstring injuries in Swedish elite sprinters

and jumpers: a pro- spective randomised controlled clinical trial comparing two reha- bilitation protocols. Br J Sports Med. 2014;48(7):532–9.

10. Dubois B, Escalier JF. Soft-tissue injuries simply need PEACE and LOVE. Br J Sports Med. 2020;54(2):72–73. https://doi.org/10.1136/bjsports-2019-101253. Epub 2019 Aug 3.

11. Mendiguchia J, Martinez-Ruiz E, Edouard P, Morin J.-B, Martinez-Martinez F, Idoate F, and Mendezvillanueva A, Multifactorial A. Criteria-based Progressive Algorithm for Hamstring Injury Treatment. Med. Sci. Sports Exerc. 2017;49(7):1482–1492.

12. Edouard P, Richardson A, Murray A, Duncan J, Glover D, Kiss M, Depiesse F, Branco P. Ten tips to hurdle the injuries and illnesses during major athletics championships/practical recommendations and resources. Front Sports Active Living. 2019;1:12.

13. Edouard P, Mendiguchia J, Guex K, Lahti J, Samozino P, Morin JB. Sprinting: a potential vaccine for hamstring injury? Sport Perf Sci Rep. 2019;48:v1.

Athletics: Throwing

5

Giacomo Zanon, Enrico Ferranti Calderoni,
Alberto Polizzi, Alessandro Ivone,
Eugenio Jannelli, and Franco Benazzo

5.1 Characteristics of the Sport

The most important sports in track and field throwing sports are hammer, shot put, javelin, and discus. Despite the international popularity of throwing events, few studies have been reported and our knowledge is lacking in this area. They are some of the most ancient sports in history: the shot put and the discus were part of the first modern Olympic game in 1896, hammer was added in 1900, and javelin in 1908. Moreover, throwing sports are the most common sports among girls and are second only to football for boys' sport in high school [1]. Throwing athletes generate very high forces over a short period,

during the kinetic chain, repetitive stress could be a source of throwing injuries. Improving the knowledge about biomechanics events and about the mechanism of throwing injuries leads to a conscious involvement in terms of prevention, diagnosis, treatment, and rehabilitation strategies. Because of the difference between the mature and the immature skeleton, including bone plasticity and epiphyseal growth plates, different risk factors should be studied [2]. The kinetic chain activation allows the energy, which come from the feet on the ground, to run through the legs, the pelvic ring, the trunk, and the throwing arm. In other words, the kinetic chain scheme is made of different steps which represent the linkage of multiple body segments providing activation, mobilization, and stabilization for transfer of forces and motion. Every throwing event requires a specific technique; otherwise, they share the same scheme of the kinetic chain. This is the reason why throwing sports share common injuries; conversely, the difference aspects of the kinetic chain and of risk factors lead to distinct injuries. Abduction and external rotation represent the common aspects: the shoulder represents one of the most involved sites of injury in throwing events [1].

G. Zanon (✉)
Responsabile Sport Medicine Surgery, Habilita Group,
Clinica ortopedica dell'Università degli Studi di Pavia,
Fondazione IRCCS Policlinico San Matteo, Pavia, Italy
e-mail: zanon.g@libero.it

E. F. Calderoni · A. Polizzi · A. Ivone · E. Jannelli
Dipartimento di Ortopedia e Traumatologia,
Fondazione Policlinico IRCCS San Matteo,
Università di Pavia, Pavia, Italy
e-mail: e_ferranti@libero.it

F. Benazzo
Sezione di Chirurgia Protesica ad Indirizzo
Robotico - Unità di Traumatologia dello Sport,
U. O Ortopedia e Traumatologia Fondazione
Poliambulanza, Brescia, Italy
e-mail: francesco.benazzo@poliambulanza.it

5.2   Physiological and Biomechanical Demands on Athletes

5.2.1   Hammer

The hammer is a metal ball which is attached to a handle by a steel wire. The weight is 7.3 kg for men and 4 kg for women. The beginning phase is determined by arm swings followed by three to five turns with the hammer extended horizontally to obtain the maximum angular acceleration. Each rotation has a component of both single and double support. Only during the final turn of the double support phase, the hammer can achieve acceleration. For this reason, coaches and throwers have sought to extend the duration spent in double support. Shifting the center of mass enables the thrower to maintain balance, opposing the centrifugal force created by the rotation that exceeds the weight of the athletes. The angle of flexion of the knee, the relationship between angles of torque of the hips and shoulders and the height of the hammer at release contribute at the final result. Finally, there is the release phase [1].

5.2.2   Shot Put

The athlete throws a metal ball of 7.26 kg for men and 4 kg for women in a throwing circle of 2.135 m. The rotational and the glide are two different techniques used to put the shot. The first one is more complex than the glide and requires more coordinated footwork. The purpose is to build up rotational inertia, which is maximized by using a long sweeping motion of the free leg. During the spin, the upper body is rotated opposite the lower extremities creating a wide hip shoulder separation. This builds torque by stretching the core muscles, which store potential energy to be transferred through the arm to the shot for release. In the first phase of the glide technique, the athlete makes their way from the back to the front of the throwing circle, driving with the nondominant leg. For a brief portion, the athlete is airborne while the back foot is momentarily lifted off of the ground. During this phase,

the lower body generates significant force while the upper body is relatively passive. In the power position, the dominant leg touches down first, followed by the nondominant leg. The upper body remains back and passive, with the shot held over the back leg and close to the body while the nonthrowing arm is held back behind the thrower's body. The front leg braces against the toe board with significant force as the throwing motion is initiated. As the throwing arm begins its motion in a forward arm strike, the elbow moves from a flexed to extended position while the shoulder remains adducted. The front hip remains behind the knee to promote maximum blocking as both legs extend. During the final release, both legs lift off the ground. Biomechanics studies have shown that for optimal performance, the release angle should be between 31 and 36°. In both the glide and rotational techniques, building energy through the lower extremities while keeping the body back creates the effect of loading a spring; the potential energy is transferred as kinetic energy through the upper extremity and to the shot for release [1].

5.2.3   Javelin

Javelin throwing technique consists of five phases. The first component is the approach where the thrower runs in the direction of the throw to build momentum. The second phase is a series of sideways crossover steps, stretching the trunk and throwing muscles. The third component is the transition from running to throwing of the athletes. The fourth phase is determined by the javelin release when the athlete comes to an abrupt stop, transferring momentum from forward motion of body to forward motion of javelin in an overhead throwing motion. Finally, in the last component, the thrower regains balance after deceleration of the throwing motion. Glenoid labrum, the glenoid ligaments and the anterior joint capsule stabilize the glenoid from anterior translational forces when the arm is abducted and externally rotated. The muscles of the rotator cuff along with the long head of the bicep tendon contribute to the dynamic stabilization. The follow through phase generates the greatest muscle contraction and joint forces after the release of the implement; all muscle groups are active as eccentric contraction of muscles slows down the arm. To increase the distance range over which force may be applied to the javelin, throwers achieve high shoulder external rotation while limiting shoulder internal rotation during the approach run and crossover. The repetitive internal rotation of the glenohumeral joint will lead to tightening of the rotator cuff in the posterior capsule. Repeated eccentric stresses on the rotator cuff with eccentric loading and excessive external rotation can cause microtrauma of the rotator cuff tendons [1].

5.2.4 Discus

The discus is 220 mm in diameter and weighs 2 kg for men and 181 mm and 1 kg for women. It is gripped with palm and fingers and thrown after several rotations as the athlete moves toward the front of a 2.5-m circle. The throw consists of five phases: initial double support, single support, flight, second double support, release and delivery. The first phase starts with double support which is the time between maximum backswing and right foot takeoff. This marks initiation of the traverse across the circle, where the trunk is rotated, loading the core muscles to optimize torque potential, and both arms are extended to provide counterbalance of the reduction in base support. The second phase is the single support one when the left foot takes off as the body moves into single support on the right leg. The arms remain extended and the trunk rotated to promote maximum potential and kinetic energy as the right foot takes off and the body rotates. The body is then accelerated forward during flight phase. The thrower lands on the right foot, which plants and pivots. The body leans forward and knees are bent to lower the center of mass. The left foot then plants, moving the thrower into second double support phase where the body is perpendicular to the direction of the throw. Following the second double support phase there is the release one that is characterized by release of transfer of stored energy into the discus through

the kinetic chain. The body rotates toward field first through the pelvis, then the trunk, the chest, and the throwing arm. Finally, the delivery phase, characterized by the final release of the discus, should be released between 35 and 40° [1].

5.3 Epidemiology

Throwing sports injuries represent 5.9% of boy's and 6.7% of girls' track and field traumatic events in American high school while 20% of all track and field injuries in Swedish elite athletes, with no statistically difference between female and male. The percentage of throwers who sustained at least one injury throughout their career is 70%, and more than 28 days of training were missed in 40% of throwers. Shot put is considered the most dangerous among throwing sports, with an incidence of injuries of 2.9% for males and 3.6% for females of all track and field injuries. According to D'Souza et al., 46% of traumatic events are located in the ankle, which is considered the most common site of injuries. Particularly in shot put where the toe board is used as a break for the lead leg after moving forward at high velocity and can determinate inversion and rotational forces of the ankle. Moreover, cases of osteoarthritis of midfoot and ankle due to repetitive microtrauma are presented in literature. Finally, ankle twist can occur on landing after a flight phase in discus and shot put. Excessive rotatory forces to the knee are also associated with ACL anterior cruciate ligament (ACL) and meniscal tears, such as in shot put, discus, and hammer throws. The back is involved instead in 31% of injuries in throwing athletes. Heavy loads on the axial structures are associated with hyperextension and rotation of the lumbar spine. According to Schmitt et al., several cases of retired javelin throwers are described with spondylolysis and spondylolisthesis, which is more than in the general population. Moreover, lumbar muscle strain and spondylarthrosis are highly common in shot put and discus throwers. Another important body part interested is the shoulder (70% of upper extremity injuries), which is particularly susceptible to rotator cuff disease due to repetitive stress and to some anatomical features. According to Rathbun et al., some areas are less vascularized and therefore are predisposed to injuries. During the most abducted and externally rotated phase of throwing the supraspinatus, infraspinatus, teres minor, and latissimus dorsi are most involved. The rotator cuff also has to oppose to distraction, horizontal adduction, and internal rotation during the deceleration of the arm after release [1]. MRI scans of 21 javelin throwers retired with an average of 19 years (range 10–25 years) after the end of performance showed osteophytes or sclerosis in the caudal, ventral, and dorsal zones of the glenoid fossa and in the cranial, caudal, and ventral zones of the head of the humerus. Complete ruptures of the supraspinatus tendon of the rotator cuff were seen in five patients, while complete ruptures of the infraspinatus or teres minor tendon in one case. In 13 shoulders (65%), the supraspinatus was affected by partial tears, and in 16 shoulders (80%) the external rotators. However, only a few felt handicapped. This phenomenon is well known as limited mobility seldom causes pain and can be overcome by compensatory movements of the shoulder-girdle. Repetitive trauma can also determine degenerative changes, such as capsular laxity and increased external rotation range of motion and decreased internal rotation range of motion [3]. According to Thorsness et al., the long head biceps tendon (LHBT) and superior labrum is an important site of injury in elite javelin throwers. SLAP tear is the most common form of superior labrum lesion, especially type II SLAP tears. Compression, distraction, and throwing or overuse have all been implicated in the SLAP pathology. In a recent study, it has been demonstrated that an increased horizontal abduction beyond the coronal plane of the scapula during the late cocking phase results in higher contact pressure between the posterior superior glenoid and the articular side of the rotator cuff, which may potentially lead to SLAP lesions or rotator cuff tears. Moreover, a weak subscapularis muscle may contribute to the peel back mechanism of SLAP lesions [4]. In javelin throwers, in the late cocking phase of throwing, the maximal abduction external rotation position of the arm leads the labrum and the biceps tendon to displace medially. The pathology of shoulder internal impingement is attributed to excessive and repetitive contact of the greater tuberosity and the posterior–superior glenoid. This leads to impingement of the posterior–superior cuff and labrum. Shot putters are also vulnerable to latissimus dorsi and teres major tears during release due to their explosive activation. Elbow injuries represent 15% of upper extremity trauma accidents. They are extremely common in javelin throwers subject to important valgus forces during the late cocking phase and early acceleration when the shoulder is externally rotated and the elbow is flexed. The ulnar collateral ligament (UCL) is the most important stabilizer of the elbow. Particularly, the anterior bundle resists valgus stress while the elbow is flexed from 30 to 120°. Repetitive traumas can lead to a medial pain, incompetence, and valgus instability. Moreover, microruptures of the medial capsula tendon lead to calcifications and in the sequel raised lateral pressure against the capitulum causes cartilaginous damages. With UCL insufficiency, flexor carpi ulnaris and the flexor digitorum profundus that represent dynamic stabilizers of the elbow during valgus stress, are prone to injury. Heavy valgus stress can also lead to the acutely ruptured UCL with avulsion of the medial epicondyle. The literature describes some cases of ulnar neuropathy in javelin throwers associated with repetitive and significant valgus stress. The wrist and the hand are less involved at 7% of all upper extremity injuries. Particularly vulnerable to these kinds of injuries are shot putters, where the wrist is required to produce a forceful flick in an extended position during the release of the weight. Intersection syndrome is a tenosynovitis of the extensor tendon sheaths and is a common lesion in shot putters due to repetitive wrist extension that causes friction between the intersection of extensors of the thumb and wrist. Other important injuries are strains and tears of the wrist flexors. Hyperextension injuries of the long finger are common in throwers if the release of the implement (with the exception of the hammer) is not optimal. Full or partial volar plate rupture at the proximal interphalangeal joint with or without an avulsion fractures can occur with long finger hyperextension deformity [1].

5.4   Rehabilitation and Return to Play

Rehabilitation treatment for a shoulder injury aims to restore full ROM, strength, static and dynamic stability, neuromuscular control, and decrease the risk of reinjury. Rehabilitation consists of four phases: acute, intermediate, advanced strengthening, and return to throwing. In the acute phase of rehabilitation, the main aim is to restore function. Protection from further injury, restoration of ROM, reduction of pain and inflammation (using anti-inflammatory medication or various injection), and possible initiation of closed kinetic chain exercises are the first treatment goals. During the intermediate phase, the purpose is to restore functional strength, increase sport specific strength and endurance, continue full pain-free ROM, and optimize neuromuscular control. In the advanced strengthening phase, the aim is to begin open kinetic chain exercises and increase sport-specific strength and endurance. Finally, the return to-throwing (RTT) phase consists in a sport specific program of full strength, pain-free, emphasizing neuromuscular and proprioceptive control and flexibility. Thrower's Ten Exercise Program and the Advanced Thrower's Ten Exercise Program are specific rehabilitative programs for throwing athletes. The Thrower's Ten focuses on strength training and stretching exercises, while the Advanced Thrower's Ten exercise program focuses on neuromuscular control, strength, coordination, endurance, and muscular balance. The rehabilitation program following debridement or labrum repair of SLAP lesion depends on the severity of the pathology and other concomitant procedures. Arthroscopic debridement is usually performed in types I and III SLAP lesions, and the goal of the rehabilitation treatment is to restore ROM rapidly because the biceps-labral anchor is stable and intact. Between the seventh and tenth postoperative weeks (depending on the extent of concomitant tears) the athlete returns to gradual sport-specific activities. Conversely, a type II SLAP lesion is repaired by suture anchors and the purpose of the rehabilitation program is to ensure that forces and loads on the repaired labrum are appropriately controlled. Moreover, a type II SLAP repair may be associated with arthroscopic plication, capsular shift, or Bankart repair. Therefore, the patient should sleep in a shoulder abduction sling for the first 4 weeks following surgery and full ROM should be obtained within 12 weeks. To prevent stiffness secondary to elbow injuries, the rehabilitation should focus on an early range of motion program using a brave to avoid valgus overload, strengthening, and a gradual throwing program. However, it is preferable to prevent high elbow flexion levels in the first period of rehabilitation. In fact, a cadaver study demonstrated that elbow flexion at $90°$ produces more UCL strain than at full extension to $50°$ of elbow flexion. According to Udall et al., both the flexor digitorum superficialis and flexor carpi ulnaris play important roles in the valgus stability of the elbow. Moreover, UCL rehabilitation protocols should incorporate strengthening of these muscles. A specific postoperative program after UCL reconstruction does not exist for javelin throwers. Hoverer, according to Dines et al., the mean return to the throwing program was 8 months after surgery to increase strength in the forearm and shoulders and to prevent reinjuries. The return to competition, conversely, was 15 months [5]. Most upper and lower extremity injuries can be managed nonoperatively with oral analgesics, activity modification, and rehabilitation. Conversely, surgical intervention is proposed for shoulder and elbow recalcitrant cases and rare traumatic ruptures. According to the literature, the pathology involving the biceps–labrum complex leads to a difficult return to a preinjury level, although most cases do not separately identify overhead athletes. Only 55% of athletes with posterior instability return to their preinjury level of competition after posterior capsule–labral repair, although 89% of throwers reported good or excellent results on clinical outcomes. Repetitive microtrauma in an overhead athlete's shoulder can lead to anterior instability due to the attenuation of the anterior soft tissue. A possible consequence of anterior micro instability can be glenohumeral internal rotation (GIRD), which is associated with posterior capsular tightness, partial undersurface rotator cuff tears, and SLAP lesions, and the primary care is a nonoperative treatment. Stretching of the posterior–inferior capsular leads to 90% of athletes returning to play, but there is a lack of high-level studies validating outcomes for the surgical management with capsular release. Controversial results are obtained in overhead athletes subjected to operative treatment for type II SLAP lesions. However, a recent systematic review demonstrated that 64% of patients return to their preinjury level after SLAP repair, with rates as low as 7% when evaluating overhead athletes. Therefore, biceps tenodesis can be used as a solution in patients with SLAP tears and coexisting biceps tendinitis with good clinical results. Chalmers et al. also demonstrated that athletes who undergo open biceps tenodesis have more physiologic pitching mechanics when compared with athletes who undergo SLAP repair, evaluating the differences between neuromuscular control and upper extremity motion during the overhead pitch. Electromyographic measurements submit altered patterns of thoracic rotation in athletes who had undergone SLAP repair. Moreover, the natural muscular activation pattern within the long head of the biceps was better restored in patients treated with tenodesis than SLAP repair. Popeye deformity and potential for biceps muscle cramping postoperatively are a contraindication to perform a tenotomy in overhead athletes. Finally, labrum debridement achieved good outcomes and prevents the possible alteration of ROM. According to Martin and Garth, in fact, 87.5% of athletes with isolated anterior or posterior glenoid labral tears treated with debridement obtained excellent results and 67% of throwers returned to priori level of play. Unsatisfactory surgical outcomes are obtained in throwing athletes with rotator cuff tears. While 76% of overhead athletes with partial thickness rotator cuff tears treated with surgical debridement were able to return to play, only 55% returned to their preinjury level. Full-thickness rotator cuff tears in overhead throwing athletes have the worst prognosis following repair. Mazoue and Andrews evaluated 14 professional overhead athletes with full-thickness rotator cuff tears at a mean follow up of 66 months, and only two players were able

to return to play at preinjury level. Nonoperative treatment remains the initial treatment for elbow medial UCL partial injuries and severe tears in most recreational throwers. However, surgical repair and reconstruction of UCL have obtained satisfactory outcomes. Suture and drill holes were used to repair 40 humeral MUCL and 11 ulnar MUCL after failure of a minimum 3 months of rehabilitation. Good and excellent results were reported in 93% of patients and 58 of 60 athletes returned to the same level of sports by 6 months after surgery. Conversely, 10 javelin throwers were evaluated with a minimum of 2 years of follow up after reconstruction of UCL and 100% of the patients were subjectively satisfied with their clinical outcomes [4].

5.5   Prevention Strategies

An adequate prevention has to be focused on risk factors and characteristic of the track and field throwing sports. Due to biomechanics complexity, prevention demands more attention than before and has to be investigated with more studies. Prevention is classified into primary subgroup, including athletes without injury during they activity, and secondary subgroup which consists of throwers with injury in their medical history or signs of fatigue. Repetitive stress, also during training, increases the risk of injury. An appropriate balance must be achieved between practicing to achieve consistent form but minimizing repetitions to prevent overuse. Moreover, flexibility is frequently not considered as important when talking about track and field throwing sports, for example, dynamic stretching is preferable to static exercise. Moreover, the data shows that the quality of equipment is quite relevant to prevent injury. Some studies focused on quality of foot plant, which is critical to maintain biomechanics, particularly in throwing sports involving rotation phases. In addition, the track has to be dry and flat to avoid slipping, sprain, or wrong stress. According to Terzis G. et al. [6], multiple studies have demonstrated a correlation between muscular strength and performance in track and field throwing sports. Throwing athletes spend a significant portion of their time in strength training, and this provides another opportunity for injury. The majority of these kinds of tears depend on the relationship between repetitive stress and the shortness of recovery time. Schmitt H. et al., suggest that long-term changes in throwing arm occur due to the duration of high-performance phase and training with weights of more than 3 kg. This explain the importance to achieve a balance between the right technique, using preventive training units (i.e., stimulation with light weights such as elastic bands), and sufficient recovery time. Trakis et al. [7] found a relevant difference between throwing and nonthrowing arm in a group of adolescent throwers with medical history of shoulder pain. The supraspinatus and the trapezius seem to be weaker and the intrarotatory muscle group stronger in throwing arm instead of nonthrowing arm. The prevention protocols should be focused on the muscular imbalance; in other words, they have to include posterior muscle strengthening. Moreover, some data collected in a cadaver lab show a reduction of internal impingement due to the strengthening of the subscapularis muscle. According to D'Souza et al., the importance to achieve an appropriate technique is proved: establishing a long-lasting partnership with a trainer who works with the athletes every day to improve their skills, also during competition, is a positive predictor in terms of injury risk [1].

References

1. Meron A, Saint-Phard D. Track and field throwing sports: injuries and prevention. Curr Sports Med Rep. 2017;16(6):391–6.
2. Mautner BK, Blazuk J. Overuse throwing injuries in skeletally immature athletes-diagnosis, treatment, and prevention. Curr Sports Med Rep. 2015;14(3):209–14.
3. Schmitt H, Hansmann HJ, Brocai DR, Loew M. Long term changes of the throwing arm of former elite javelin throwers. Int J Sports Med. 2001;22(4):275–9.
4. Thorsness R, Alland JA, McCulloch CB, Romeo A. Return to play after shoulder surgery in throwers. Clin Sports Med. 2016;35(4):563–75.
5. Wilk KE, Macrina LC. Nonoperative and postoperative rehabilitation for injuries of the throwing shoulder. Sports Med Arthrosc Rev. 2014;22(2):137–50.
6. Terzis G, Stratakos G, Manta P, Georgiadis G. Throwing performance after resistance training and detraining. J Strength Cond Res. 2008;22(4):1198–204. https://doi.org/10.1519/JSC.0b013e31816d5c97. PMID: 18545188.
7. Trakis JE, McHugh MP, Caracciolo PA, Busciacco L, Mullaney M, Nicholas SJ. Muscle strength and range of motion in adolescent pitchers with throwing-related Pain: implications for injury prevention. Am J Sports Med. 2008;36(11):2173–8. https://doi.org/10.1177/0363546508319049.

Basketball

6

Tassery François, Daniele Mozzone, Groc Mariane, Pascal Edouard, and Patricia Thoreux

6.1 Characteristic of the Sport

6.1.1 Introduction

Basketball was invented in 1891 in the United States. Basketball is an Olympic team sport in which two teams of five players compete on an indoor court of 28 × 15 m, according to the rules of the International Basketball Federation (FIBA:http://www.fiba.basketball/OBR2017/Final.pdf). The goal is to score points by throwing the ball into the hoop of the opponent located at a 3.05 m height from ground level.

The game is played in four quarters of 10 (FIBA) or 12 (NBA) minutes each, and it cannot end in a tie. When the two teams have the same score at the end of the regular time, one or more overtime periods of 5 minutes are played until one of the two teams prevail. A recent practice has emerged called "three-by-three" basketball (3 × 3). In this sport, two teams of three players compete on an outdoor half-court, with synthetic surface flooring. This sport was on the program of the Tokyo 2020 Olympics (https://tokyo2020.org/en/games/sport/olympic/basketball/). It is currently the second most practiced team sport in France.

With the collaboration of: Allaire A, Allaire T, Bouvard M, Chermann J-F, Colle J, Dannel B, Delagarde J-C, Foshia C, Garcia S, Giraudeau N, Guincestre J-Y, Labruyere C, Le Ho M, Lhotellier D, Moraux A, Rodineau J, Rouch P, Tassery B.

T. François
Fédération Française de Basket—FFBB (Medical Commission), Paris, France

D. Mozzone
Federazione Italiana Pallacanestro—FIP (Youth National Teams Department), Torino, Italy

Istituto di Medicina dello Sport di Torino FMSI, Torino, Italy

G. Mariane
Département Médical de l'INSEP (Institut National du Sport, de l'Expertise et de la Performance), Paris, France

P. Edouard
Unité de Médecine du Sport, Service de Physiologie Clinique et de l'Exercice, Hôpital Nord, CHU Saint-Etienne, Saint-Etienne, France

Laboratoire Inter-Universitaire de Biologie de la Motricité (LIBM EA 7424), Université Jean Monnet, Université de Lyon, Saint-Etienne, France

P. Thoreux (✉)
Département Médical de l'INSEP (Institut National du Sport, de l'Expertise et de la Performance), Paris, France

CIMS (Centre d'Investigations en Médecine du Sport), Hôpital Hôtel Dieu—APHP, Paris, France

Institut de Biomécanique Humaine Georges Charpak—Arts et Métiers Paris Tech—Université Sorbonne Paris Nord, Paris, France
e-mail: patricia.thoreux@aphp.fr

The physiological demands in basketball have been assessed in numerous studies: it requires approximately 1000 different movements per game, with direction and rhythm changing every 2–3 s, including 105 sprints (8% of match time) with an average duration of 1.7 s. Other types of movement include tramping and lateral movements (especially during defense phases) for 31% of match time, fast races for 12%, slow races for 11%, walking or standing periods for 35%, and an average of 45 jumps per game (3% of game time). Players perform an average of 5–6 km and 45 jumps per game. Each player per match is exposed to an average of 8 impacts superior to 5G per minute explaining the numerous traumas which can occur. Top basketball players have VO2max values around 45–50 ml/min/kg and the average heart rate during a match is approximately 90% of the maximum heart rate, highlighting the intensity of this sport. In 3 × 3 basketball, the smaller court results in lower HRmax values (83% of HR max), but intensity and changes in pace and direction appear to be more important. There are physiological differences between 5 × 5 basketball and 3 × 3 basketball, which are both Olympic sports. According to Montgomery and Maloney [1], the characteristics of 3 × 3 significantly highlight the anaerobic sector: the intensity of a match is doubled in 3 × 3, and the 3 × 3 players have aerobic abilities that are 25% lower than the 5 × 5 players. The differences could be due to the total distance run per match (4500 m traveled in 5 × 5 vs. 870 m to 1470 m in 3 × 3).

Basketball has changed over the years, and nowadays, the game is more physical, with more contact between players. This is accentuated by their impressive physical characteristics: for high-level masculine players, the average height is 200 cm and average weight is 95 kg. These elements combined with the rhythm and the efforts developed by the players make basketball a high-risk sport for injuries, which can be non-contact and contact injuries.

6.1.2 Epidemiology of Injuries in Basketball [2, 3]

A recent study by Foschia et al. [3] summarized the epidemiology of acute injuries in basketball already published. They gathered the data from 21 articles for a total of 46.504 basketball players and 20.175 injuries and reported an overall incidence of 5.7 injuries per 1000 h of practice, and 13.0 injuries per 1000 athlete-exposure; this represented approximately 7.7 injuries per season per team.

Regarding the location of injuries, the lower limbs are by far the most affected location (64% of total injuries), followed by the upper limbs (14%), the head (10%), and the trunk (9%). The ankle is the primary location of lower limbs (40%), followed by the knee (26%). Sprain is the main type of injury (39% of all injuries), followed by muscle contusions (18%), acute musculotendinous injuries (16%), and chronic tendinopathies (12%). An ankle sprain, which is mostly lateral, is the most frequent diagnosis in basketball players (16% of all injuries), followed by finger sprains or dislocations (13%), muscular lesions of the thigh (quadriceps or hamstrings) (11%), and knee sprains (8.5%). In knee injuries, anterior cruciate ligament rupture is responsible for 44% of so-called surgical injuries and 36% of so-called severe injuries requiring more than 30 days of interruption of sporting activity.

Being male, over 20 years of age, professional, and at high-level seem to be risk factors associated with injuries. The most-at-risk playing positions are the points guards, accounting for 41% of all injuries, followed by small and power forwards (36% of all injuries), and centers (22% of all injuries).

Injuries can be classified from minor to serious according to the time needed for the return to play.

Minor injuries require less than a week for the return to competition, while serious injuries range from mild (less than 2 weeks) and major (up to 5 weeks) to severe (more than 5 weeks).

Most injuries, roughly 80% of all cases, lead to a quick return to play, generally within a couple of weeks.

Approximately 20% of all injuries can be classified as serious, with the ankle having the highest rate of serious injuries, followed by calf lesions.

Ankle and knee sprains are the most common and the most studied type of injury, but we would rather focus on slightly less common and often underestimated pathologies, such as the traumatic concussion, the dental trauma, the patellar tendinopathy, and the ankle retinacula pathologies.

6.2   Concussion [4]

Over the past 15 years, concussion has become one of the most challenging traumas.

Major advances have been made in the prevention of concussions and especially in their diagnosis. Basketball is considered a non-risk sport for concussion. However, literature data, mainly from the North American basketball leagues, show a significant number of concussions. Moreover, a concussion protocol has been implemented in the NBA since the 2011–2012 season. This has enabled a great improvement in the protection of the athletes.

In 2016, we undertook an initial inventory of concussions in French basketball (FFBB) with the objective of also setting up a concussion protocol. This epidemiological study, based on a questionnaire, was carried out with all the French national basketball teams (EDF) in 2017 (358 athletes). Of the 220 responses (62%), 10.4% reported having suffered from concussion in their career. We found a loss of consciousness in approximately 40% of cases and a post-concussion syndrome in 40%.

In 2019, a new descriptive epidemiological study with individual interviews conducted by a sport physician trained in concussion was published. It confirmed the presence of concussions in high-level basketball with a prevalence of 24% in the same population (EDF). In this study, pre-season tests were also conducted, which included SCAT 5, as well as neuropsychological tests such as Trail Making Test (TMT A and B), Digit Symbol Test, and a test on the Neurotracker Virtual System. These tests can be used as a reference in case of a concussion for the return to play protocol. These tests should also be able to track the cognitive status of players over the seasons in search of a possible cognitive decline that may be correlated to a cumulative number of concussions. These two studies (unpublished data)

enabled sportsmen, coaches, assistants, physical trainers, medical and paramedical staff, and sports organizations to be more aware of the issues related to concussions in high-level French basketball.

Subsequently, the Federal Medical Commission of the FFBB has established a regulatory protocol for the management of concussion for the 2019/2020 season. For the elite Jeep and Pro B (competitions organized by the National Basketball League) a referring "concussion" physician is officially appointed to each team, whose decision is notified to the match commissioner. If there is suspicion of concussion, the referee will stop the game and request the intervention of the referring doctor to perform the Maddocks score FFBB*. If the player does not answer one question correctly, he will be taken out of the game and attended to by the physician for a more accurate medical assessment. It is the doctor's responsibility to determine when to allow the player back in the match. The referee will record the concussion protocol on the match sheet and the player's eventual return to the game. At the end of the match, the referee will send a report to the LNB Medical Committee and will give the player and his relatives a fact sheet "what to do in case of concussion."

For competitions organized by the FFBB (French Championship level), a doctor is not always present. The referee will signal the suspicion of concussion and will request the intervention of the player's coach to carry out the Maddocks score. In the event of an incorrect answer, the player will be taken out of the game and may only come back under the sole responsibility of his team (coach, leader, or doctor if present). The referee will record the concussion protocol on the match sheet which will also be signed by the player's coach. A report will be sent to the Federal Medical Commission and a fact sheet "what to do in case of concussion" will also be given to the player and his relatives.

*Maddocks score FFBB version** (1. In what city/arena are you playing in today? 2. Where is your team playing today? 3. What team are you playing against? 4. Which team did you play against in the last game? 5. Did your team win the last game?).

6.3   Dental Trauma

There is a classification, established by the International Dental Federation, of sports with dental traumatic risk. Basketball has a high incidence of oral trauma.

A study published in the ADA journal, based on dental trauma claims from 1996 to 2005 at the Athletic Department of Southern California University in Los Angeles, shows that basketball has the highest rate of dental injuries. This study shows a risk five times higher than in American football.

A survey conducted in 2017 by S. Garcia, MD and the University of Montpellier, France, showed that 43% of basketball players from National Teams had already seen other players suffering from a dental trauma, and 28% of them had already suffered a dental trauma themselves.

Oral traumas can be divided into two major categories: soft tissue traumas (gums, cheeks, lips, tongue) and hard tissue traumas (teeth, alveolar bone and maxillary bone).

From the laceration of the lips to the fracture of the maxillary bone bases and the expulsion of one or more teeth, the consequences on the time of the return to play are very variable.

An open lip requires the player to leave the court immediately in order to stop the bleeding. This situation can be time-consuming in the short term, but generally without long-term impact. A fracture of the mandible means the athlete cannot play for several weeks, like for example Brandon Jennings (basketball player) in 2015 or Henry Immelman (rugby player) in 2018, out of game respectively 3 and 6 weeks.

In addition to the consequences for the staff and the club, the athlete himself is the first to suffer the consequences of his trauma. Several measures, such as nutritional restrictions over a short or long period and special monitoring must be adopted to avoid any adverse development, such as the formation of an oral infection, which may itself be responsible for other disorders affecting performance. The replacement of a lost tooth following a trauma can sometimes require multiple operations: bone grafts, gum grafts, dental implant, and others.

Factors that increase dental trauma risk include untreated cavities, periodontal disease, badly positioned wisdom teeth, and other dental alignment disorders.

The best mean of prevention is the intraoral custom-made protection (mouth guard), made by a dental technician under the supervision of a dental surgeon. The adaptable protections found in sport's shops can sometimes cause more harm than good.

6.4   Patellar Tendinopathy [5]

6.4.1   Epidemiology and Risk Factors

In basketball, tendinous pathologies are most frequent, due to the repetition of jumps and landings, i.e., by plyometric and eccentric work. Its incidence is estimated at 2.7/1000 h of practice in a Dutch group of basketball players of all levels.

It is estimated at 7% among 14–18 year olds at high level, 32% among 19–29 year olds, and 45% of professional basketball players.

Intrinsic and extrinsic risk factors for patellar tendinopathy have been identified in basketball players.

The major extrinsic risk factor is over extensive training.

According to Ferreti, the risk of patellar tendinopathy increases with the number of hours of training: 2 training sessions /week: 3.2%; 3 training/week: 14.6%; 5 training/week: 41.8%.

Tendon constraints are major during jumps (6–10 times the body weight). The maximum stress peak appears on landing.

According to Benitez-Martinez et al. [5], most professional basketball players have abnormalities of the patellar tendon: 91 tendons/146 have abnormalities (73 players), 28.8% of players have only one abnormal tendon, 48% of players have a bilateral abnormality, and 23.2% of players have no abnormalities.

There is no influence of the dominant side.

There are many intrinsic risk factors: age, height, overweight, genetic factors, flexibility, static disorders, muscle strength, neurosensitivity and motor control, etc.

For example:

- The risk in men is due to the greater power of their quadriceps, while women would more likely develop patellar tendinopathy due to insufficient quadriceps muscles (especially in the eccentric range).
- Decreased dorsal ankle flexion (the after-effect of an ankle sprain) increases the possibility of developing patellar tendinopathy.
- A failure of neuro-muscular control has an influence on torso stability and lower limb movements.

6.4.2 Diagnosis

Pain, amplified by effort, is anterior topography (patella tip, tendon body, proximal part).

The functional impact is assessed by the VISA.P score and/or by the Blazina, Roels, or Martens Classification.

Clinical examination includes the classic triad: pain on palpation, contraction, and stretching.

Assessment of static disorders of the lower limbs is necessary: feet, knees, hip, and spine.

Isokinetic assessment to evaluate the muscular strength of the quadriceps and hamstrings and especially the quadriceps eccentric/quadriceps concentric ratio can be performed.

Functional assessment can be made by jump tests (Myotest) coupled with video.

6.4.3 Ultrasound is the Reference Exam

From an anatomic standpoint, patellar tendon should be considered as a ligament rather than a tendon because it joins two bones. It is a fibrous broad band 3–5 mm thick, fibrous and hyperechoic, inserted proximally on the apex of the patella and distally on the anterior tibial tuberos-

ity. Repetitive microtrauma may lead to morphological changes of the tendon leading to tendinopathy.

Patellar tendinosis most commonly involves the proximal insertion of the tendon.

On sagittal US images, the tendon will appear thickened with a fusiform hypoechoic thickening on its deep central portion at its insertion on the patella. On transverse US images, the hypoechoic thickening appears as a round hypoechoic nodule with a posterior bulging of the central and deep fibers of the tendon.

Intratendinoushyperhaemia is usually depicted in power Doppler or color Doppler imaging.

Central tears and calcifications may be encountered in chronic tendinopathy.

6.4.4 Treatment

The treatment should be preventive as the first episode, and its management influences the subsequent development of recurrent tendonitis. It includes reinforcement of the torso, stability and alignment of the lower limbs, neurosensitivo-motor reprogramming exercises and stretching.

Curative treatment includes rest from sports, physiotherapy care (physiotherapy, radial shock waves, etc.), adapted rehabilitation (eccentric, HSR, etc.).

6.4.5 Conclusion

The treatment of patellar tendinopathy must be managed by a team effort involving the player, medical staff, and technical staff as patellar tendinopathy with structural damage only allows recovering of the function but not the full healing of the tendon.

6.5 Ankle and Retinacula

The pathology of the retinacula is poorly understood. The damage to these structures is varied

and accompanies or complicates many pathologies (ankle sprains) that cause chronic
symptomatologies.

The dynamic nature of ultrasound is useful for
detecting their possible disintegration.

6.5.1 Anatomical Reminder

Retinacula are aponeurotic thickeners that
strengthen or duplicate superficial aponeuroses.
They have bone anchorage points that make them
firmly adhere to the cortex and especially to the
periosteum.

The retinacula are composed of 3 layers: the
most peripheral is formed by a vascularized connective tissue, the middle layer consists of transverse fibers of collagen and elastin and the medial
layer constitutes the sliding surface where we
find longitudinally oriented collagen fibers and
fibroblasts.

Their role varies with their topography:

- If their role relates to the strengthening of the
aponeurosis, their purpose is to maintain a
structure in place, most often a tendon that
remains pressed against the cortex, which prevents it from "taking the rope" in the event of
muscle contraction.
- If their role is to duplicate an aponeurosis, we
observe the formation of a tunnel that not only
holds the structure (tendon or vasculo-vascular
nerve) in place but also serves as a "guide" to
this structure.

6.5.1.1 Topography
The anatomy and also the pathology of the retinacula of the foot and ankle are the most complex, and therefore, the most unknown.

6.5.1.2 Retinacula Pathology

The Types of Injuries
In the acute or sub-acute stage, partial or total
ruptures and disinsertion are observed, but also
disbonding.

In the chronic stage, thickening either partially or completely is essentially observed.

The Different Retinacular Pathologies of the Foot and Ankle
- Disbonding lesions are observed when the
tendons of the fibular lateral and posterior
medial tibial tendons are dislocated; these
lesions, often unknown clinically, may be
accompanied by the tearing off of a bone
flake. Particular attention must be paid to this
and the residual thickening because, in the
vast majority of cases, the tendon recovers
after the acute episode and only the dynamic
test (contraried eversion in lateral and contraried inversion in medial) affirms the diagnosis. These movements must therefore be
systematically performed during an ankle
ultrasound and in particular in the assessment
of a sprain. This disbonding may also be partial, not leading to a real tendon malposition
causing a reactive thickening of the insertion
area.
- Breaks are rare. The cases observed are injuries by direct trauma to the dorsal side of the
tarsus.
- Desinsertions are more frequent and often
unknown; they can concern the retinaculum of
the extensors, which then take the "rope" and
move further away from the tibia on the
injured side during the dorsal flexion of the
ankle. Lesions, always partial, can also be
detected at the insertions of the extensor retinaculum at the superficial part of the sinus of
the tarsus and at the calcaneal attachment of
the lower fibular retinaculum, causing atypical
pericalcanineal pain.
- Insertion enthesopathies, linked to repeated
tensile phenomena, are found at all retinacular
attachments, particularly at the perimalleolar
level but also at the medial attachments of the
retinacula of the flexor tendons.

The most common semiological element is
retinacular thickening which is reactive to many
etiological factors. On the dorsal side of the tarsus, some athletes (especially basketball players)
experience disseminated increases in the thickness of the retinacula of the extensors, suggesting
repeated traction phenomena. In addition, tendon
ruptures, tendinopathies and peritendinopathies

may lead to an increase in the adjacent retinaculum. The conflicts by extrinsic friction (with the shoe or a splint) that are sometimes at the origin of disseminated increase should also be noted.

Apart from retractions, stenotic phenomena can result from these thickenings. It is the tendons that are most often enclosed in these clamp-like positions which limit their mobility and are a source of secondary tenosynovitis.

6.5.1.3 Conclusion

The pathology of the ankle and foot retinacula is very varied and polymorphic. Some lesions predominate according to their topography and must be systematically looked for. If not, an inaccurate diagnosis might be made and could lead to incorrect treatment.

Total or partial ruptures are post-contusional lesions but can also result from excessive traction.

High-resolution ultrasound plays a crucial role in the dismemberment and follow-up of lesions. This is the best technique to clarify the pathological role of these structures.

6.6   Rehabilitation and Return to Play [6]

In modern sport, rehabilitation and return to play are a team process involving the team physician, the physiotherapist, the athletic trainer, the coach, and last but not least the injured player.

A sport psychologist should also take part in the process, as many injuries may have profound mental consequences on the athlete, and the mental approach can positively or negatively affect the recovery phase.

The final aim is allowing the safest and quickest return to play to the athlete, reducing the risk of re-injuries.

The team physician and physiotherapist take care of the early rehabilitation, far from the basketball court.

Painkillers and NSAIDs prescription is widespread, and their use may have a role in helping the physiotherapist to start the treatment as soon as possible.

When the acute phase is over and the athlete has regained strength, full mobility, balance and agility, the athletic trainer takes charge of the athlete for the sport specific on field re-conditioning necessary before the return to play.

When the player is able to run at high intensity, jump with no discomfort, perform swift changes of direction, dribble and shoot, he can be considered ready to join the team again. During the first few practices, it is necessary to progressively increase the volume and intensity of exercise, starting with the warm-up and the no-contact drills, and then increasing the length and the work load.

If everything is fine, the player can get the final clearance to take part in the whole training session and then in the game.

Because many minor or overuse injuries do not necessarily endanger or prevent a player from practicing or playing a game, the constant communication between the team physician, the technical staff, and the player itself is of the utmost importance, to constantly monitor the athlete problem, immediately detect any signs of deterioration in his conditions and decide if, when and for how long it is necessary to stop him or limit some of the sport activities.

6.7   Prevention Strategies [7]

Most studies focus on the assessment of preventive measures to protect the players from two of the most frequent and severe injuries: the ankle sprain and the ACL rupture.

Talking about ankles, the strongest risk factor for an ankle sprain is having suffered from a previous ankle sprain, along with other factors such as poor balance control and limited ankle range of motion. For this reason, primary prevention is fundamental. The strategies that granted a significant protection against this kind of injury, or at least resulted in less severe ankle sprains, are the implementation of a neuromuscular training program, the use of taping, and of ankle braces.

Ankle braces result to be more cost effective and easier to apply than tape.

The neuromuscular training program consists in a series of exercises that improve proprioception and balance.

High-top shoes were not found to be safer than low-top shoes. The stability of the foot inside the shoe appears to be more important than the shoe height in the prevention strategy.

Talking about ACL, many risk factors were discovered, including the female sex, anatomic factors such as the increased slope of the tibial plateau, a decrease of the intercondylar femoral notch size and an increased antero-posterior knee laxity, a decreased neuromuscular control and a prior ACL reconstruction among others.

Unfortunately, no prevention program was actually shown to reduce the risk of this kind of injury in basketball, unlike in many other multi-directional sports such as soccer, volleyball, or hand ball where similar programs proved to be effective.

Preventing overuse syndrome is a matter of balancing the work load of the training sessions with the resting time, considering the age and the level of the players.

Stretching and muscular eccentric exercise may be very useful to increase the mobility of the joints and strengthen muscles and tendons, to increase the body tolerance to the relevant athletic requests of this sport.

The French Basketball Federation has developed a prevention approach, including clinical follow-ups, isokinetic tests, video coupled jump tests, Visa P, patellar tendon ultrasounds and tendon elastography, and dental check-ups.

To be effective, the players, medical staff, and technical staff must fully adhere to the suggested protocols.

References

1. Montgomery PG, Maloney BD. Three-by-three basketball: inertial movement and physiological demands during elite games. Int J Sports Physiol Perform. 2018;13:1169–74.
2. Andreoli CV, Chiaramonti BC, Biruel E, de Castro Pochini A, Ejnisman B, Cohen M. Epidemiology of sports injuries in basketball: integrative systematic review. BMJ Open Sport Exerc Med. 2018;2018:4(1).
3. Foschia C, Tassery F, Cavelier V, Rambaud A, Edouard P. Les blessures liées à la pratique du basketball: revue systématique des études épidémiologiques. J Traumatol du Sport. 2019;36(4):242–60.
4. McCrory P, Meeuwisse W, Dvorak J, Aubry M, Bailes J, Broglio S, Cantu RC, Cassidy D, Echemendia RJ, Castellani RJ, Davis GA, Ellenbogen R, Emery C, Engebretsen L, Feddermann-Demont N, Giza CC, Guskiewicz KM, Herring S, Iverson GL, Johnston KM, Kissick J, Kutcher J, Leddy JJ, Maddocks D, Makdissi M, Manley GT, McCrea M, Meehan WP, Nagahiro S, Patricios J, Putukian M, Schneider KJ, Sills A, Tator CH, Turner M, Vos PE. Consensus statement on concussion in sport—the 5th international conference on concussion in sport held in Berlin, October 2016. Br J Sports Med. 2017;51(11):838–47. https://doi.org/10.1136/bjsports-2017-097699.
5. Benıtez-Martınez C, Valera-Garrido F, Martınez-Ramırez P, Rıos DJ, Bano-Aledo ME, Medina-Mirapei F. Lower limb dominance, morphology, and sonographic abnormalities of the patellar tendon in elite basketball players: a cross-sectional study. J Athl Train. 2019;54(12):1280–6. https://doi.org/10.4085/1062-6050-285-17. by the National Athletic Trainers' Association, Inc.
6. Malanga GA, Chimes GP. Rehabilitation of basketball injuries. Phys Med Rehabil Clin N Am. 2006;17(3):565–87.
7. Taylor JB, Ford KR, Nguyen AD, Terry LN, Hegedus EJ. Prevention of lower extremity injuries in basketball: a systematic review and meta-analysis. Sports Health. 2015;7(5):392–8.

Cycling

7

Kazumi Goto and Jacques Menetrey

7.1 Characteristics of the Sport

The remarkable feature of cycling is its high-speed and to be performed in peloton with a minimum of protective equipment. Physiologically, cycling is one the most demanding sports with an extremely heavy training load and repetitive back to back and stage competitions. Another characteristic is that races are held under various weather conditions. All these features exposed athletes to a high risk of traumatic and overuse injuries. Although there are various disciplines in cycling, the combined risks are common to all kinds of cycling. The different characteristics of each type of cycling are summarized in Table 7.1.

Table 7.1 The characteristics of cycling disciplines

Type	Specificity
Road bicycle race	Competition for running power on the road
	The race distance ranges from a few kilometres to 300 km
Track bicycle race	Competition for running power on a special runway
	The race distance ranges from a few hundred meters to several thousand meters
Mountain bike race (MTB)	Race mainly on unpaved roads using special bicycles called mountain bikes
	There are several types of competitions (downhill, cross-country, marathon)
Cyclo-cross	Competition on land such as forest roads, pastures, sand, and field with zone of portage
Bicycle motocross (BMX)	Competition on a course or space with many undulations such as artificially constructed jump tables and turns

7.2 Physiological and Biomechanical Demands on Athletes

Cycling is physiologically extremely demanding. It requires heavy training loads and discipline. It is a sport of sacrifices. Races last from a few minutes to 7 h and energy expenditure can reach up to 7500 kCal/day. The repetitiveness of efforts in stage races is unique in the world of sports. Cycling requires strength, balance, and coordination. Technique in cycling can be assessed through measurement of joint kinematics and

K. Goto
Centre for Sports Medicine and Exercise, Swiss Olympic Medical Center, Hirslanden Clinique la Colline, Geneva, Switzerland
e-mail: kazumi@kgorthop.com

J. Menetrey (✉)
Centre for Sports Medicine and Exercise, Swiss Olympic Medical Center, Hirslanden Clinique la Colline, Geneva, Switzerland

Orthopaedic Surgery Service, University Hospital of Geneva, Geneva, Switzerland
e-mail: Jacques.Menetrey@hirslanden.ch; jacques.menetrey@hcuge.ch

muscle activation patterns. When the bicycle is optimally fitted, the range of motion of the joint is as follows. Hip: flexion from 28° to 90°, Knee: flexion from 37° to 111°, Ankle: extension of 53 to 103° plantar flexion (neutral position defined as 90°). If you regard the pedalling cycle as a circle, it can be divided into two stages. The stage of 0° (when pedals are at the top of crank position) to 180° is called a power phase and 180° to 360° is a recovery phase. In power phase, gluteus maximus and vastii group (quadriceps) works mainly from 315° to 105°, while hamstring work from 45° to 200°. Vastii group and hamstring are both active for 70° of crank movement. Within the recovery phase, iliopsoas and rectus femoris work together. Gastrocnemius and soleus muscles activate after the hip and knee extensors, ranging from 27° to 145° for the soleus and from 35° to 260° for the gastrocnemius, making it the muscle with the longest period of contraction during the pedal stroke cycle.

7.3   Epidemiology of Injuries

Injuries can be classified as traumatic or overuse lesions according to their mechanism. Several studies are reported about the epidemiology in road racing. It has been shown that traumatic injuries accounted for 40–54% of all injuries in top-level cyclist (Fig. 7.1).

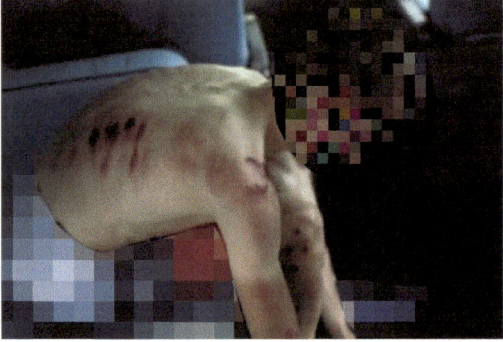

Fig. 7.1 "Road rash" is an occupational hazard for cyclists who cause interference at some stages. It is a wound caused by friction as you slide along the road or track. The epidermis, the top layer of the skin, is removed. Depending upon the severity, some underlying layers may also be removed

Regarding traumatic injury, the most common lesion was skin abrasion/laceration (59–67%). The incidence of fracture was reported as 21–27%. The most commonly fractured bones were the clavicle (17–27%), wrist (6–12%), and rib (3–8%) [1].

Overuse lesions were more frequent in professional cyclists. Overuse injuries include musculoskeletal, perineal, and genital complaints. The most common musculoskeletal overuse injuries reported differed in each study. Barrios et al. reported that the most frequent lesion was tendinopathy, located around the knee in 17–29% and at the Achilles' tendon in 8–15% [2]. Clarsen et al. investigated overuse lesions in 109 cyclists of seven professional teams over one year. In this study, lower back pain (58%) and anterior knee pain (36%) were the most prevalent problems.

Professional road cycling has undergone a major transformation not only under the form of technical advances in race bicycles but also with the application of new training protocols and the best of sports science, and finally, with a spectacular increase in competitiveness over the past decade. These changes should also affect the epidemiology and the characteristics of injury occurring in cycling competitions. The rate of traumatic injuries in elite cyclists had nearly doubled from the 1980s and early 1990s to the period 2003–2009 [2]. In a recent study, the epidemiology of injury, operative incidence, and return-to-competition timeline were evaluated among 1584 elite cyclists competing in the Tour de France over a span of 8 years. Injuries had a major impact on .cyclists, with 16% of athletes withdrawing because of an injury each year. A total of 138 withdrawals were caused by acute trauma, 49% of which were fractures, which represented the most common reason for withdrawal. A total of 29 (43%) riders with fractures underwent surgery.

Concussion is one of the most severe injuries in cycling trauma in general. The report in the USA showed that approximately 1.4 million persons were treated for mild trauma brain injuries annually in the USA and, out of these, an estimated 207,830 were related to sports and recreation. Cycling was reported to account for 40,424 (19%) of the cases, the highest number in any sport. As noted in previous

Table 7.2 Previous reported data of world class top cyclists with traumatic injuries [2]

Diagnosis	1983–1995 65 cyclists	2003–2009 66 cyclists
Total number	**34**	**76**
Clavicle fractures	9 (26.5%)	13 (17.1%)
Laceration/contusion	8 (23.5%)	13 (17.1%)
Wrist fractures	4 (11.8%)	9 (11.8%)
Craniofacial fractures	2 (5.9%)	4 (5.3%)
Hip fractures	3 (8.8%)	3 (3.9%)
Ribs fractures	1 (2.9%)	5 (6.6%)
Muscle ruptures	1 (2.9%)	4 (5.3%)
Meniscus tears	1 (2.9%)	3 (3.9%)
Spine fractures	1 (2.9%)	2 (2.6%)
Knee ligament ruptures	0	2 (2.6%)

Table 7.3 Previous reported data of world class top cyclists with overuse injuries [2]

Diagnosis	1983–1995 65 cyclists	2003–2009 66 cyclists
Total number	**52**	**65**
Patellofemoral pathology	15 (28.8%)	4 (6.1%)
Patellar tendinopathy	10 (19.2%)	8 (12.3%)
Mechanical low back pain	7 (13.4%)	9 (12.8%)
Achilles tendinitis	8 (15.4%)	5 (7.6%)
Iliotibial band syndrome	2 (3.8%)	9 (12.8%)
Paraspinal cervical muscles contracture	0	7 (10.6%)
Hamstring contracture	0	6 (9.1%)
Quadriceps tendinopathy	4 (7.7%)	0
Quadriceps contracture	0	4 (6.1%)
Lumbar disc herniation	0	3 (4.6%)
Triceps contracture	0	2 (3.0%)

reports, the incidence of head injuries was 1.3–10% of all injuries reported during cycling events. Moreover, concussion requiring less than 48 h of inpatient observation was reported as 2%, and this incidence is increasing (Tables 7.2 and 7.3).

7.4 Rehabilitation and Return to Sport

The detailed protocol of rehabilitation and return to sport for traumatic or overuse injuries associated with cycling would depend upon the nature of the lesion. According to the aforementioned study about the Tour de France, the time to return to competition varied widely (7–316 days). The mean time to return to competition for cyclists whose withdrew because of an injury was 52 days compared with a mean return-to-competition time of 32 days for cyclists who withdrew for non–trauma-related reasons. Overall, 43% of fracture injuries required surgery, and those undergoing surgery had a longer time to return to competition (77 days) versus for those treated non-surgically (44 days) [3]. However, the time to return to competition from clavicle fractures treated operatively was significantly shorter compared with the same injury treated nonoperatively. While further details characterizing the fracture pattern are necessary, the operative fixation of clavicle fractures may allow for a quicker return to competition.

Because concussion is a life-threatening trauma, deep knowledge in terms of return to play is required. First of all, obtaining an assessment of the cyclist's baseline neurologic function is one of the most important steps of good neurological care. Establishing a baseline neurological function allows for a more accurate diagnosis in case of future injury and helps guide for their safe return to cycling. Cyclists who have a history of prior concussion are at an increased risk of repeat injury; therefore, it is particularly imperative for these cyclists to have a baseline cognitive and motor control assessment performed prior to the start of the racing season. Now, the most challenging task for the team staff is to assess a concussed rider during a race. Often, the rider victim of a concussion is going back on their bike as long as they are willing and able to ride. However, they can suffer from slower reaction time and impaired information processing speed, placing themselves and the peloton at risk for further injury [4]. On field SCAT-5 assessment and Maddock's questions can be used in race conditions. However, Maddock's questions have been validated in a team sport setting (e.g., football, ice-hockey, rugby, basketball), and more appropriate questions would be required for cycling. One recent systematic review [4] suggested alternative road cycling specific Maddock's questions such as:

1. What is the name of this race?
2. How many kilometers are there still to go in today's stage?
3. Who is the road captain today for the race?
4. What was your last race?
5. What is your coach's name?

These questions could be asked through the radio by the team Doctor, but road cycling specific questions should be further developed with the Union Cycliste Internationale (UCI) in collaboration with the medical staff of teams.

7.5 Prevention Strategies

To prevent cycling injury, it is important to know the general mechanism of traumatic and overuse injury. We should also pay attention to issues such as strength and flexibility imbalances and technical errors. In addition, bad bicycle fitting is one of the major causes of cycling overuse disorders; thus, appropriate adjustment is necessary as a prevention strategy.

Traumatic injury can occur as a combination of several factors, not just a single factor, including poor infrastructure, road conditions, mechanical failure, operator error, and vehicle interaction. During the race, competitors are in close proximity and running at high speeds, which can cause mechanical failure and accidental contact such as wheel contact and/or shoulder clash. Therefore, racers must be skillful, stay calm, and show respect to their peers. Anticipation of obstacles and headset are also part of the preventive program. Union Cycliste Internationale (UCI), the governing body of competitive cycling in the world, requires the use of approved helmets in all racing events. Cyclists significantly decrease their odds of head and skull injury by wearing helmets, but helmets cannot prevent concussion yet.

In addition to bike fitting, one of the most important factors to prevent overuse injury is hip abductor muscle strength. Although not specific to cycling, it has been reported that gluteus medius insufficiency is correlated with lateral ankle sprain, patellofemoral pain, iliotibial band (ITB) friction syndrome, and anterior cruciate ligament injury. The hip abductor affects the biomechanics of the lower limbs by stabilizing the pelvis and preventing excessive torque around the knee. Furthermore, several studies demonstrated that core stability should reduce the risk of injury [5]. On the basis of observational studies, delay in activation or weakness of the core muscles is related to low back pain and lower extremity injury [6]. Interventions should aim at restoring core stability in order to prevent overuse injuries in cycling.

It has also been reported that anterior knee pain is related to bicycle settings [7]. It is usually caused by a low or forward saddle position, or an excessively long crank, and/or an increase in knee flexion at the top of the pedal stroke leading to an increase in the patellofemoral contact pressure. Incorrect width between the feet and the pedals relative to the hips has also been reported to cause anterior knee pain. Rotational deformation should also be addressed during bike fitting and proper pedals should be set on an individual basis.

References

1. Barrios C, Bernardo ND, Vera P, Laíz C, Hadala M. Changes in sports injuries incidence over time in world-class road cyclists. Int J Sports Med. 2015;36(3):241–8. https://doi.org/10.1055/s--0034-1389983. Epub 2014 Nov 6
2. Clarsen B, Krosshaug T, Bahr R. Overuse injuries in professional road cyclists. Am J Sports Med. 2010;38:2494–501.
3. Haeberle HS, Navarro SM, Power EJ, Schickendantz MS, Farrow LD, Ramkumar PN. Prevalence and epidemiology of injuries among elite cyclists in the Tour de France. Orthop J Sport Med. 2018;6(9):81–2.
4. Elliott J, Anderson R, Collins S, Heron N. Sports-related concussion (SRC) assessment in road cycling: a systematic review and call to action. BMJ Open Sport Exerc Med. 2019;5:e000525.
5. Asplund C, Ross M. Core stability and bicycling. Curr Sports Med Rep. 2010;9(3):155–60. https://doi.org/10.1249/JSR.0b013e3181de0f91.
6. Leetun DT, Ireland ML, Wilson JD, et al. Core stability measures as risk factors for lower extremity injury in athletes. Med Sci Sports Exerc. 2004;36:926Y34.
7. Kotler DH, Babu AN, Robidoux G. Prevention, evaluation, and rehabilitation of cycling-related injury. Curr Sports Med Rep. 2016;15(3):199–206. https://doi.org/10.1249/JSR.0000000000000262.

Extreme Sports

8

Francesco Feletti and Omer Mei-Dan

8.1 Characteristic of the Sports

With millions of participants worldwide, extreme sports (ESs) are profoundly transforming sports participation, and many of them have been recently recognized as Olympic disciplines.

For example, over the past two decades, snowboarding, mountain biking, and BMX racing were included in the Olympic programs, kiteboarding made its first appearance in the Olympic arena at the 2018 Youth Olympic Games in Buenos Aires and to be included in the 2024 Paris Olympic Games. Surfing, sport climbing, BMX freestyling, and skateboarding debuted at the 2020 Olympic Games in Tokyo, while ski-mountaineering will be Olympic at Milano-Cortina 2026.

ESs can be defined as activities involving unusual physical and mental challenges such as speed, height, depth, or natural forces, where an unsuccessful outcome is likely to result in injuries or death [1].

Indeed, the perception of risk associated with these activities determines the idea that people have of the participants. At the same time, most athletes participating in ESs recognize that their sports involve significant risks.

However, sports participants invest a considerable amount of time and commitment in preparation to reduce these risks [2]; and there is evidence that, to some extent, ESs are not riskier than traditional sports activities.

For example, in climbing sports, the injury incidence and severity score is lower than in many traditional sports, such as sailing, basketball, and soccer, while the death rate reported among climbers in the UK (1:4000) is significantly lower than that reported for motorcycle riding (1:500) [3, 4].

The available epidemiological data are too sparse and fragmented to extend these conclusions to the entire domain of ESs; however, ESs represent the fastest growing area among sporting activities this century, and more emphasis could be put on their positive characteristics rather than on risk.

Apart from risk, some specific traits highlight ESs compared to more traditional sports, including the role of environment-related variables, the use of hi-tech equipment, and their spectacular-

F. Feletti (✉)
Department of Diagnostic Imaging, S. Maria delle Croci Hospital, Ausl Romagna, Ravenna, Italy

Dipartimento di Medicina Traslazionale e per la Romagna, Università degli Studi di Ferrara, Ferrara, Italy
e-mail: feletti@extremesportmed.org

O. Mei-Dan
Department of Orthopedics, School of Medicine, University of Colorado, Aurora, CO, USA

© The Author(s), under exclusive license to Springer-Verlag GmbH, DE, part of Springer Nature 2022
G. L. Canata, H. Jones (eds.), *Epidemiology of Injuries in Sports*,
https://doi.org/10.1007/978-3-662-64532-1_8

ity, which results in an influential appeal to fashion.

Moreover, the benefits of ESs might be prominent over the perceived negative aspects.

For example, participation in ESs can enhance the uptake of physical activity and can improve resilience, self-worth, self-control, and environmental awareness [5].

Even if reduced to a minimum, a certain amount of injuries must be considered an unavoidable counterpart of the beneficial aspects related to sports activities.

Knowledge of the epidemiology of injuries related to ESs can guide the diagnosis, treatment, and rehabilitation of injuries sustained during their practice.

Moreover, such data may be essential to allow participants and governing bodies to develop relevant sport-specific safety policies concerning equipment, training, protective clothing, and other safety systems, design sport-specific safety guidelines, and steer future safety research.

Compared to traditional sports, the injury mechanisms and the pattern of injury of ESs are less understood, particularly the pattern of injury in many sports.

Theremore, the purpose of this chapter is to discuss the physiological and biomechanical demands on athletes, review the epidemiology of injuries in ESs, and highlight some peculiarities of prevention strategies.

8.2 Physiological and Biomechanical Demands on Athletes

ESs involve components of adventure, the danger of physical harm, and excessive levels of physical exertion. Such elements result in tremendous physical demands and stress on the body's physiological systems.

From the physiological point of view, ESs may be broadly categorized into two groups: sports involving extreme mental stress and ultra-endurance activities.

Participation in many ESs causes a high reactivity to stress within the endocrine system; indeed, according to the available literature, high circulating levels of catecholamines, growth hormone, prolactin, and cortisol are found during or soon after sports practice.

On the other hand, in those ESs of a prolonged endurance nature, such as ultramarathons, some physiological changes occur to adjust cardiovascular, metabolic, and immunological functions required for physical performance.

Each sport has specific patterns of movement and biomechanics and includes different phases of execution, styles, or disciplines, which are also distinguished in terms of physiological demands. As a matter of fact, in many ESs, the most popular discipline is freestyle, a free combination of jumping tricks and evolutions. Freestyle is commonly intercalated with phases of simple traveling, also called *crossing*, which has completely different physiological demands.

For example, in kitesurfing, freestyle requires an intense activity involving both aerobic and anaerobic metabolism. At the same time, the *crossing* is a principally aerobic effort, characterized by a considerable increase in blood pressure and heart rate due to the isometric contraction of the large muscle masses of the trunk and lower limbs [6, 7].

Some ESs are practiced in hostile environments characterized by extreme environmental-related aspects, such as humidity, temperature, and pressure, which can play a primary role in the physiology of ES.

For example, in alpine sports, such as mountaineering, physiological changes related to high altitude are among the main pitfalls and may result in altitude illness (21.3% above 2,500 m) [8] such as acute mountain sickness, high altitude pulmonary edema, and high altitude cerebral edema.

At the opposite end, scuba diving involves unique challenges associated with the changes in pressure that occur during descent and ascent through the water column. More generally, extreme watersports require immersion in a liquid with a high thermal conductivity that is frequently cold.

Finally, ultra-endurance activities such as mountain running, skyrunning, and endurance running expose participants to changes in body water composition, and the risk of electrolyte imbalances is strongly influenced by climatic conditions such as temperature and humidity level.

8.3   Epidemiology of Injuries

ESs have specific dynamics of injury, which may result in different anatomic distributions and types of injuries, as reported in Table 8.1.

The characteristic mental attitude of participants strongly influences epidemiological research in ESs. For example, minor injuries such as ankle sprains, knee sprains, lacerations, or bruises are widespread in BASE jumping, but are not reported because most jumpers do not consider them real injuries.

Some ESs-related orthopedic injuries are sport-specific; for example, the tenosynovitis of the wrist extensor tendons is a typical overuse injury in the control hand of kayakers, while flexor tendon pulley ruptures and lumbrical shift syndrome are specific for the sport of climbing [2].

"Skier's thumb" refers to the rupture of the ulnar collateral ligament (UCL) of the thumb's metacarpophalangeal joint (MCPJ) caused by trauma while handling the ski pole, "Skimboarder's toe" indicates hyperdorsiflexion injuries of the metatarsophalangeal joint associated with skimboarding, while the fracture of the lateral process of the talus is referred to as "Snowboarder's fracture".

8.4   Rehabilitation and Return to Sport

The management of ESs-related injuries is a challenge to surgeons and sports physicians because participants are inclined to return to their sports practice, irrespective of their functional outcome.

Moreover, most ESs require an "all-or-nothing" level of performance, and a gradual return to sport is not possible.

Finally, the resumption of sport in sub-optimal conditions may result in life-threatening injuries rather than merely reinjury, as in the case of more traditional sports [2].

Some general principles should be taken into account when approaching the rehabilitation of an ESs athlete.

It is generally essential to overtly recognize with the athlete that injury rehabilitation will be a stressful period.

It may be essential to involve other stakeholders, such as the coach, in order to arrange realistic timeframes for a return to sport. Some ESs participants may exhibit over adherence to rehabilitation, and empowering them with the awareness of their deficits, as well as the use of a rehabilitation diary, may help develop proper adherence to rehabilitation.

Recovery from an injury in ESs entails consideration of injury etiology, pain mechanisms, pathology, tissue healing, and mediating athlete-specific functional impairments with sport-specific demands.

Functional stability or optimal neuromotor control are required; therefore, the proprioceptive component of rehabilitation is crucial in addition to muscular strength, power and endurance.

Core stability, balance training, plyometric exercise, co-contraction exercises, and rhythmic stabilization should be integrated and progressed from the beginning.

Exercises with a reduced base of support or destabilizing equipment (e.g., Bosu ball, physio-ball, trampette, dura disc) may be preferred to include the proprioceptive challenge [10].

In order to facilitate specific motor learning, rehabilitation should include the repetition of sport-specific exercises that replicate the functional stances, strength, and agility demands of each activity.

Representation or simulation of the experience of sporting activity helps the athletes to link the restoration of movement schemes and the following sporting technique. Using a pool to prac-

Table 8.1 Epidemiology of Injuries in the most popular extreme sports [2, 9–11]

Sport	Injury rate[a]	Dynamics of acute injuries[b]	Anatomic location of injuries (%)[b]	Most common injuries (%)[c]
Indoor climbing [12]	0.027–0.079/1000 hours	• Fall resulting in wall or ground strikes	Fingers (41) Forearm/elbow (13.4) Foot (9.1)	Flexor tendon pulley rupture (45) Tenosynovitis (15.5) Joint capsular damage and ligament injuries (13.6) Fractures (3.3)
Rock climbing [12]	0.2/1000 hours	• Jamming of a hand/finger in a crack or pocket hold • Loss of a foothold resulting in sudden additional stress on a hand		
Ice climbing [12]	2.87–4,07/1000 hours	• Falling ice	Head (47.6) Knee (14.3) Shoulder (11.9)	Open wounds (52) Hematoma (20.6) Frostbite (8.8) Fractures (1.9)
Mountaineering [8]	0.005–0.013/hours/person	• Slip on snow or ice • Fall • Rock fall	Leg (36.9) Head (20.9) Multiple (16.7)	Fractured tibia (10.7) TBI (12) Multiple abrasion contusion (9.4)
Alpine Skiing [13]	1–2/1000 participant days	• Direct impact with the snow surface or obstacles • Collision with ski edges • Falls onto an outstretched hand	Knee (33.4) Head/face(13.5) Shoulder (9.5)	Sprain/strain (47.7) Fracture (18.9) Contusion (12)
Snowboarding [13]	2–4/1000 participant days	• Off-balance falls	Wrist (24.9) Head/face (14.3) Shoulder (13.1)	Fracture (35) Sprain/Strain 25.9) Contusion (12.7)
Skydiving [14]	48–170/100,000 jumps	• Landing miscalculation, (e.g. low turn, landing off headwind) • Parachute opening deceleration	Lower limbs (51) Upper limbs (19) Spine/back (18)	Fracture (54.3) Contusion (20.6) Sprain/strain (15.4)
BASE Jumping [15]	2/1000 jumps	• Object strike, bad landing	Lower limbs (61) Spine/back (20) Chest wall injuries (18)	Fractures (81.5) Multi trauma (5.5) Concussion (3.7)
Whitewater canoeing and Kayaking [16]	4.5–5.2/paddler days	• Extreme bracing or support strokes	Upper extremities (61) Head/face (16)	Sprains (35) Tendonitis (20) Fractures (23)
Rafting [17]	0.26–0.44/paddler days	• Collisions with other rafters, impacts from paddles, entanglement of extremities with the raft	Face (33) Knee (15) Shoulder (6)	Lacerations (33) Strains/sprains (23) Fractures (23)
Surfing [18]	4/1000 surfing days	• Contact with the surfboard • Contact with the seafloor • "Wiping out" by the wave	Head/face (18–49) Lower extremity (6–32)	Lacerations/abrasions (35–46) Sprains/strains (12–39) Fractures (5–16%)
Kite surfing [19]	7/1000 hours	• Cuts/bruises caused by contact with sharps edges, kite lines or rocks • Falls from intentional jumps • Loss of control over the kite	Ankle/foot (28.2) Trunk (16.1) Head (13.7)	Laceration/Abrasion (47.3) Contusion (33.8) Joint sprain (9.7) Fractures (3.2)

Table 8.1 (continued)

Sport	Injury rate[a]	Dynamics of acute injuries[b]	Anatomic location of injuries (%)[b]	Most common injuries (%)[c]
Wakeboarding [20, 21]	12/1000 hours	• Falls due to unpredictable disturbances such as the bow wave of the boat or natural obstacles • Landing from a ration jump over an artificial obstacle • ACL rupture is mainly caused by landing with the flat undersurface of the board against the water in an axial loading type mechanism	Head (47.9) Hip and lower extremity (26.5) Shoulder and Upper Extremity (14.8)	ACL rupture (31) Lacerations to the head/neck (24.6) Shoulder dislocations (14.7) Fractures (10.1)
Snow kiting [22]	8.4/1000 hours	• Mismanaged execution of high jumps • Collisions with obstacles • Collisions with other snowkiters	Trunk (21.7) Head (15.2) Shoulder/arm (15.2)	Contusion (32.7) Joint sprain/Muscle strain (23.9) Laceration/abrasion (17.3) Fractures (4.3)
Kite buggying [23]	Unknown	• Kite lifting the athlete out of the buggy ("out of buggy experience") • Lifted by kite while not on the buggy • Flipped buggy	Spine (18) Thorax (18) Shoulder (23)	Vertebral fractures (15.4) Rib fractures (17.9) Shoulder dislocations (10.2) Fractures (66)
Skateboarding [24, 25]	7–7.5/1000 participants	• Falls due to loss of balance and irregularities in the riding surface • Failure when attempting a trick or a jump • Collision with a vehicle or an obstacle	Upper extremity (55–63) Lower extremity (17–26) Head (3.5–13.1)	TBI (36) Radius/ulna fracture (19.6) Tibia/fibula/ankle (15.4)
Windsurfing [26–28]	1/1000 sailing days	• Low-speed falls leading to "foot strap injuries" • High-speed falls and catapulting (consisting in the sailors being unable to detach the harness causing them to be launched into the air) • Causing shoulder and head injuries • Anterior shoulder dislocations are caused by the boardsailor hanging onto the boom while falling	Foot/ankle (27.8) Head (7.4) Shoulder (7.1)	Sprains (26.3) Lacerations (21.2) Contusions (16.2) Fractures (14.2)
Sailing and Yachting [29–31]	0.29–4.6/1000 days of sailing 16/1000 sailor-hours on hydrofoiling boats	• Falls on board • Collisions with fellow crew members or deck equipment • Head trauma due to moving spars • Overuse due to high-repetition activities resulting in elbow flexor/extensor tendinosis, and PINE (grinder's elbow)	Lower back (44–52.9) Knees (22–32) Head (22.1–32.4) Hand (8–31.3)	Contusions (55) Wounds (14.3–31.3) Fractures (0.4–15.1) Head Trauma (22.1)

(continued)

Table 8.1 (continued)

Sport	Injury rate[a]	Dynamics of acute injuries[b]	Anatomic location of injuries (%)[b]	Most common injuries (%)[c]
Mountain Biking [32, 33]	Recreational: 1.54/1000 h. Downhill 16.8/1000 h.	• Lost control on soil in poor trail conditions • Accidents during jumps	Calf (11.7) Forearm (10.5) Knee (8.9)	Abrasions (35) Contusion (30.8) Distortion (7.9) Fractures (3.5)
Paragliding [34]	5.8–10.1/1000 licensed pilots/year	• Collapse or deflation of the airfoil • Oversteering or pilot error • Collision with an obstacle	Lower leg (36.4) Thoracolumbar spine (24) Knee (7)	Fractures (58.3) Ligamentous injury (12.3) Concussion (2.5)
Powered paragliding [9]	6.4/1000 participants/year	• Collision with terrain/ground • Equipment malfunction • Contact with the propeller	Upper limb (44.5) Lower limb (32) Back (9.7)	Laceration/wound to the upper limb (12.1) Forearm/wrist/hand fracture (8.5) Leg/ankle/foot fracture (5.8)
Hang gliding [34]	0.007–0.08/pilots/year	• Insufficient airspeed causing pushing out or failure to control pitch attitude and angle-of-attack during takeoff • Uncontrolled landing after stalling • Falls due to turbulence and collisions	Upper limbs (22.1) Spine (19.6) Head (17.2)	Fractures (68.8) Concussion (11.4) Elbow luxation (4.9)
Mountain running, Skyrunning, Endurance running [35]	56.5% participants/competition	• Overuse • Trauma/fall • Fatigue	Knee (15–41) Lower leg muscles (13–23) Foot (16–28)	Ankle extensor tendon Synovitis of extensor retinaculum (19%) Patellofemoral syndrome (7.4–15.6) Achilles tendinopathy (2–18.5)

PINE posterior interosseus nerve entrapment, *TBI* traumatic brain injury
[a] Data resulting from studies of better quality (prospective, e.g. conducted by medical personnel) were selected and the most recent of them were preferred
[b] The three most important dynamics reported in scientific literature were reported
[c] The three most important injuries reported in scientific literature were reported and, in addition, data about fractures were always included

tice the Eskimo roll before a white water kayaker is headed to a raging river, wind tunnel practice for the skydiver, or a climbing gym workout for the alpine climber who aims for the big walls, all can be instrumental in this process.

References

1. Cohen R, Baluch B, Duffy LJ. Defining Extreme Sport: Conceptions and Misconceptions Front Psychol. 2018; 9:1974.
2. Mei-Dan O, Carmont MR. The Management of the Extreme Sports Athlete. In- Mei-Dan O and Carmont M (Eds). Adventure and extreme sports injuries. Epidemiology, treatment, rehabilitation and prevention. (Ch 1), pp 1-5. London: Springer; 2013. https://doi.org/10.1007/978-1-4471-4363-5.
3. Schöffl V, Morrison A, Schwarz U, Schöffl I, Küpper T. Evaluation of injury and fatality risk in rock and ice climbing. Sports Med. 2010;40(8):657–79. https://doi.org/10.2165/11533690-000000000-00000.
4. Storry, T. The Games Outdoor Adventurers Play. In: Humberstone BJ, Brown H, Richards K. Whose Journeys? The Outdoors and Adventure as Social and Cultural Phenomena. Penrith: The Institute for Outdoor Learning, 2003; pp. 201–228.
5. Brymer E, Feletti F. Beyond risk: the importance of adventure in the everyday life of young people. Ann Leis Res. 2020;23(3):429–46. https://doi.org/10.1080/11745398.2019.1659837.

6. Vercruyssen F, Blin N, L'Huillier D. Assessment of the physiological demand in kitesurfing. Eur J Appl Physiol. 2009;105:103–9.

7. Camps A, Vercruyssen F, Brisswalter J. Variation in heart rate and blood lactate concentration in freestyle kitesurfing. J Sports Med Phys Fitness. 2011;51(2):313–21.

8. Brustia R, Enrione G, Catuzzo B, Cavoretto L, Pesenti Campagnoni M, Visetti E, Cauchy E, Ziegler S, Giardini G. Results of a Prospective Observational Study on Mountaineering Emergencies in Western Alps: Mind Your Head. High Alt Med Biol. 2016;17(2):116–21. https://doi.org/10.1089/ham.2015.0110.

9. Feletti F, Goin J. Accidents and injuries related to powered paragliding: a cross-sectional study. BMJ Open. 2014;4(8):e005508. https://doi.org/10.1136/bmjopen-2014-005508.

10. Malliaras P, Morrissey D, Antoniou N. Rehabilitation of Extreme Sports Injuries. In- Mei-Dan O and Carmont M (Eds). Adventure and extreme sports injuries. Epidemiology, treatment, rehabilitation and prevention. (Ch 17), pp 339–361. London: Springer; 2013.

11. Laver L, Pengas IP, Mei-Dan O. Injuries in extreme sports. J Orthop Surg Res. 2017;12(1):59. https://doi.org/10.1186/s13018-017-0560-9.

12. Schöffl V. Rock and Ice Climbing. In Mei-Dan O and Carmont MR (Eds). Adventure an Extreme Sports Injuries. (Ch.2). pp 7–35. Springer-Verlag London 2013.

13. Langran M. Alpine Skiing and Snowboarding Injuries. In Mei-Dan O and Carmont MR (Eds). Adventure an Extreme Sports Injuries. (Ch.3). pp 37–67. Springer-Verlag London 2013.

14. Westman A. Skydiving. In Mei-Dan O and Carmont MR (Eds). Adventure an Extreme Sports Injuries. (Ch.4). pp 69–90. Springer-Verlag London 2013.

15. Mei-Dan O, Carmont MR, Monasterio E. The epidemiology of severe and catastrophic injuries in BASE jumping. Clin J Sport Med. 2012;22(3):262–7. https://doi.org/10.1097/JSM.0b013e31824bd53a.

16. Fiore DC, Houston JD. Injuries in whitewater kayaking. Br J Sports Med. 2001;35(4):235–41. https://doi.org/10.1136/bjsm.35.4.235.

17. Whisman SA, Hollenhorst SJ. Injuries in commercial whitewater rafting. Clin J Sport Med. 1999;9(1):18–23. https://doi.org/10.1097/00042752-199901000-00004.

18. Lowdon BJ, Pateman NA, Pitman AJ. Surfboard-riding injuries. Med J Aust. 1983;2(12):613–6.

19. Nickel C, Zernial O, Musahl V, Hansen U, Zantop T, Petersen W. A prospective study of kitesurfing injuries. Am J Sports Med. 2004;32(4):921–7. https://doi.org/10.1177/0363546503262162.

20. Baker JI, Griffin R, Brauneis PF, Rue LW 3rd, McGwin G Jr. A comparison of wakeboard-, water skiing-, and tubing-related injuries in the United States, 2000-2007. J Sports Sci Med. 2010;9(1):92–7.

21. Carson WG Jr. Wakeboarding injuries. Am J Sports Med. 2004;32(1):164–73. https://doi.org/10.1177/0363546503258910.

22. Moroder P, Runer A, Hoffelner T, Frick N, Resch H, Tauber M. A prospective study of snowkiting injuries. Am J Sports Med. 2011;39(7):1534–40. https://doi.org/10.1177/0363546511398214.

23. Feletti F, Brymer E. Injury in kite buggying: the role of the 'out-of-buggy experience'. J Orthop Surg Res. 2018;13(1):104. https://doi.org/10.1186/s13018-018-0818-x.

24. Fountain JL, Meyers MC. Skateboarding injuries. Sports Med. 1996;22(6):360–6. https://doi.org/10.2165/00007256-199622060-00004.

25. Lustenberger T, Talving P, Barmparas G, Schnüriger B, Lam L, Inaba K, Demetriades D. Skateboard-related injuries: not to be taken lightly. A National Trauma Databank Analysis. J Trauma. 2010;69(4):924–7. https://doi.org/10.1097/TA.0b013e3181b9a05a.

26. Nathanson AT, Reinert SE. Windsurfing injuries: results of a paper- and Internet-based survey. Wilderness Environ Med. 1999 Winter;10(4):218–25. https://doi.org/10.1580/1080-6032(1999)010[0218:wiroap]2.3.co;2.

27. Rosenbaum DA, Simmons B. Windsurfing. In Mei-Dan O and Carmont MR (Eds). Adventure an Extreme Sports Injuries. (Ch.9). pp189-202. Springer-Verlag London 2013

28. Arnold MP. Mountainbiken. Cooler Naturgenuss mit Nebenwirkungen [Mountain biking. Cool way to enjoy nature with side effects]. Orthopade. 2005;34(5):405–10. German. https://doi.org/10.1007/s00132-005-0791-z.

29. Schäfer O. Verletzungen beim Jollensegeln - Eine Analyse im Anfängerbereich. Sportverletz Sportschaden 2000; 14(1): 25–30. https://doi.org/10.1055/s-2000-3819.

30. Nathanson AT, Baird J, Mello M. Sailing injury and illness: results of an online survey. Wilderness Environ Med. 2010;21(4):291–7. https://doi.org/10.1016/j.wem.2010.06.006.

31. Feletti F, Brymer E, Bonato M, Aliverti A. Injuries and illnesses related to dinghy-sailing on hydrofoiling boats. BMC Sports Sci Med Rehabil. 2021;13(1):118. https://doi.org/10.1186/s13102-021-00343-8.

32. Aitken SA, Biant LC, Court-Brown CM. Recreational mountain biking injuries. Emerg Med J. 2011;28(4):274–9. https://doi.org/10.1136/emj.2009.086991.

33. Becker J, Runer A, Neunhauserer D, Frick N, Resch H, Moroder P. A prospective study of downhill mountain biking injuries. Br J Sports Med. 2013;47(7):458–62. J.

34. Feletti F, Aliverti A, Henjum M, Tarabini M, Brymer E. Incidents and Injuries in Foot-Launched Flying Extreme Sports. Aerosp Med Hum Perform. 2017 Nov 1;88(11):1016–1023. https://doi.org/10.3357/AMHP.4745.2017.

35. Park D, Carmont MR. Mountain, Sky and Endurance Running. In Mei-Dan O and Carmont MR (Eds). Adventure an Extreme Sports Injuries. (Ch.2). pp 7–35. Springer-Verlag London 2013.

Field Hockey

9

Guglielmo Torre and Rocco Papalia

9.1 Characteristics of the Sport

Field hockey is played worldwide by men and women at a recreational and professional level. It is listed among Olympic sport games and 132 national associations for field hockey exist. The International Federation of Hockey (FIH) embraces all of these associations. Although it is common opinion that this sport is less popular than others, the number of injuries sustained by players during professional competitions is significantly higher than that of professional soccer players. Field hockey is played at recreational and professional levels, with junior, men, and women categories. All continents (Europe, Americas, Africa, Asia, and Oceania) have professional leagues, promoting the sport within the nations with local tournaments and encouraging international challenges (4 Nation's Tournament, World League). The regulatory authority for all the tournaments remains the FIH.

G. Torre · R. Papalia (✉)
Department of Orthopaedic and Trauma Surgery,
Campus Bio-Medico University of Rome,
Rome, Italy
e-mail: g.torre@unicampus.it; R.Papalia@unicampus.it

9.2 Physiological and Biomechanical Demands on Athletes

Similar to the most popular sports, professionals have high requirements in terms of aerobic threshold, muscular strength, and endurance. In regular tournaments, players usually face up to six matches in one week, with average play hours between 44 and 58 min per match and a running distance between 3400 and 9500 m per match. Given the high physical and cognitive demand of athletes, the lack of an appropriate athletic endurance and preparation affects the latter game phases of the tournament, where usually the best performance is required [1]. To address this relevant issue, most of the teams adopt accurate substitution strategies, given the possibility of unlimited substitutions, to distribute the internal loads burden (physical and physiological stress) among all the players of the team. Given the high demand of running and jogging, the aerobic performance of the athlete is important in defining endurance. However, as several times running sprint or quick movements are needed, the anaerobic capacity is important as well. Therefore, the ability to recover from maximal exertion is as relevant as the capacity to cover more distance with running. Concerning musculoskeletal robustness, flexibility and stability of lower limb joints is essential for running and for changes of direction. Cutting manoeuvres and tackling are the two most risky actions that may compromise ligament integrity in knee and ankle. As muscles represents the major secondary stabilizers of knee and ankle, strengthening programs are essential to achieve good dynamic stability.

9.3   Epidemiology of Injuries

According to recent evidence in scientific literature, the rates of injury vary from 0.1 to 90.9 injuries for player-hours [2]. The number of injuries is higher during games than during training and is higher in men than woman, especially during tournaments. The main measure of "severity of injury" is the field hockey time loss. Several casuistries were reported in the literature, regarding the site of injury. The main body regions that are involved in injury are lower limbs (rate range 13–77%), head (2–50%), upper limbs (0–44%), and trunk (0–16%). Within the lower limb, most of the injuries occurred in the knee, ankle, and lower leg. Among upper extremity injuries, shoulder dislocation, clavicle fracture, olecranon bursitis, and metacarpal fractures are common. Concerning the lower limbs, groin pain syndrome, medial collateral ligament (MCL) tears (with or without anterior cruciate ligament, ACL, tears), and ankle sprains are the most common injuries. However, it has also been reported that dentofacial injury is common, with rates of 12.7% for junior players and 45.2% for elite players, with no difference in sex. However, by evaluating only tournaments of professional players, the rate of injury varies according to sex (1.2 injuries per match for men and 0.7 injuries per match). The most common types of injuries are hematomas (rate range 14–64%), abrasions and lacerations (5–51%), sprains (2–37%), and strains (0–50%). Furthermore, concussion is one of the possible injuries, although the frequency is not high (up to 25%). Non-contact injuries are the most frequent (12–64%), while contact injuries include different contact types: contact with the ball (2–52%), with the stick (9–27%), with another player (2–45%), and with the ground (9–15%). Moreover, the position within the field

was considered in a study reporting data from professional tournaments in 2013. The injuries within the circle were 50% of the total injuries occurred in women and 51% in men; injuries within the 25-yard zone were 34% of the injuries occurred in women and 32% of those occurred in men; in the midfield 12% of injuries occurred in women, and 17% of those occurred in men. Some research studies [3, 4] reported injuries by role of play, demonstrating that goalkeepers sustained the lowest number of injuries (rate range 4–19%), followed by defenders (16–36%), midfielders and forwards (22–37%).

9.4   Rehabilitation and Return to Play

Management vary significantly on the basis of the type of injury. Concussion is usually managed according to international guidelines for concussion in sports, as immediate activity stop (never allow same day continuation of training or match). Emergency department transfer for work-out is required when mental status impairment occurs. Return-to-play must be stepwise and always subordinated to complete resolution of symptoms at rest. Shoulder trauma with dislocation can be managed with on-field awake reduction, but when this is not possible, ED transfer and reduction under anaesthesia is necessary. When a single dislocation episode occurs, scapulothoracic and rotator cuff muscles strengthening program is indicated; however, multiple dislocations give the indication for surgery. After shoulder instability surgery, a recovery period of 6 months to 1 year is often sufficient for the return-to-play. Hand fractures, especially of metacarpal bones are managed according to the type of fracture. The return-to-play in these cases is allowed after complete healing of the fracture, after 4 to 6 weeks form the injury, with a short hand rehabilitation protocol after casting or splinting. Among lower limb injuries, knee and ankle sprains are the most commonly reported. In knee injuries, MCL is the commonest ligament to sustain a sprain. The clinical examination should immediately follow the trauma, as concurring swelling and muscle spasm may prevent accurate evaluation of the injury. The player should be examined out of the field, using the contralateral knee to compare stability patterns. Often, concomitant ACL tears are found and sometimes sprains of the posterior oblique ligament. The main intervention after examination consists in RICE (Rest, Ice, Compression, Elevation) and imaging work-out should follow. In those cases where surgical reconstruction is mandatory, stepwise rehabilitation protocols are used, to return gradually to full activity within 6 to 12 months.

9.5   Prevention Strategies

The International Hockey Federation has recently developed several strategies to prevent injuries and decrease the injury severity. The two main advocated strategies consist of the use of protective equipment and specific exercise training. By federal rule, goalkeepers must wear at least headgear, leg guards, and kickers. Furthermore, all players are recommended to use shin, ankle, and mouth protections [5]. Recently, mouth guards were more and more utilized during games and training sessions, with an increase of the players using them from 31.4% before 2000 up to 84.5% after 2000. Although it is strongly recommended by all regional associations to wear mouth guards, several players still do not use them. As some research studies suggested that these protections should be mandatory, some national associations have made shin, ankle, and mouth protection obligatory. Concerning exercise programs to pre-

vent injuries, it has been suggested that these should be introduced as part of the team training. Although no specific protocol of training has been already developed, exercise for the prevention of lower limb injuries are the most encouraged, as lower limbs have the highest frequency of injury. One of the most relevant strategies to prevent player fatigue is represented by substitution strategies, which allow a careful avoidance of physical overload of a single or few players. Furthermore, customized psychometric questionnaires to understand perceived levels of muscle soreness, fatigue, quality of sleep, and mood have been recently introduced, to screen players and individuate those at risk of high psychophysiological stress levels.

References

1. Ihsan M, Tan F, Sahrom S, Choo HC, Chia M, Aziz AR. Pre-game perceived wellness highly associates with match running performances during an international field hockey tournament. Eur J Sport Sci. 2017;17(5):593–602.
2. Barboza SD, Joseph C, Nauta J, van Mechelen W, Verhagen E. Injuries in field hockey players: a systematic review. Sports Med. 2018;48:849–66.
3. Theilen T-M, Mueller-Eising W, Wefers BP, et al. Injury data of major international field hockey tournaments. Br J Sports Med. 2016;50:657–60.
4. Ng L, Rosalie SM, Sherry D, et al. A biomechanical comparison in the lower limb and lumbar spine between a hit and drag flick in field hockey. J Sports Sci. 2018;36(19):2210–6.
5. Vucic S, Drost RW, Ongkosuwito EM, Wolvius EB. Mouthguard use may reduce dentofacial injuries in field hockey players. Br J Sports Med. 2016;50:298–304.

Football

10

Josè Henrique Jones, Luca Pulici, and Piero Volpi

10.1 Introduction

Football is one of the most popular contact sports in the world. Currently, FIFA unifies 211 national associations and represents approximately 300 million male and female players, who are actively involved in the game of football.

The incidence of football injuries is estimated to be 10–35 per 1000 match hours and is approximately 1000 times higher than that observed in other industrial occupations generally regarded as high risk (construction workers and miners 0.02 injuries/1000 h).

One athlete plays on average 100 h of football a year (from 50 h on amateurs' teams up to 500 in professional teams). This means that a player will have at minimum one limiting injury a year.

10.1.1 Characteristics of the Sport

Soccer is a complex sport with specific physical, technical and tactical demands. Depending on the role, different physical and technical skills are required.

It is essential to possess technical skills, which must be supported and kept constant during the game by proper physical preparation.

Being a situational sport, players need excellent cognitive skills (decision making) to make the best choice in the shortest time in relation to opponents.

10.1.2 Physiological and Biomechanical Demands on Athletes

Soccer is an intermittent sport characterized by short repeated sprints with active pauses of jogging or walking.

The total distance covered during a game depends on the role. Soccer players run between 10 km and 11 km, in some cases reaching 14 km. Approximately a quarter of this distance is covered at high intensity running.

During matches, players express efforts equal to approximately 70–80% of their Vo2 max, with heart rates around 80–90% of HRmax, and a lactate concentration of 2–10 mmol/l.

J. H. Jones (✉)
Montijo Orthopedic and Sports Medicine Clinic, Montijo, Portugal

L. Pulici
FC Internazionale Milano, Milan, Italy

P. Volpi
FC Internazionale Milano, Milan, Italy

Knee Surgery and Sports Traumatology Unit, Humanitas Research Hospital, Rozzano (MI), Italy

© The Author(s), under exclusive license to Springer-Verlag GmbH, DE, part of Springer Nature 2022
G. L. Canata, H. Jones (eds.), *Epidemiology of Injuries in Sports*,
https://doi.org/10.1007/978-3-662-64532-1_10

Continuous changes in running speed, changes in direction, movements during shots and passes are very stressful on a muscle–tendon structure; therefore, a good preparation of neuro-muscular coordination and strength is required.

Physiological demands are increasing, and thus the number of high-intensity actions and the total distance covered has increased by 30–35%, especially in European competitions.

It is important to note that the physiological and functional model in football changes according to the needs of the coach, based on tactical ideas and coach philosophy.

10.1.3 Risk Factors

In football biomechanics, three broad areas are covered: the technical performance of soccer skills; the equipment used in playing the game; and the causative mechanisms of specific soccer injuries. Kicking is the most widely studied soccer skill. In contrast, several other skills, such as throwing-in and goalkeeping, have received little attention; other skills such as passing and trapping the ball, tackling, jumping, running, sprinting, starting, stopping, and changing direction, deserve detailed biomechanical investigation.

The external factors such as equipment, boots, the ball, artificial and natural turf surfaces, shin and mouth guards are always updated during investigation. Some soccer injuries may be related to the equipment used or surfaces.

Climate and environmental factors of different geographical regions play an important role in performance and injury risk. Football injury risk seems to increase with increased age, career duration and previous injury. Mechanical instability in ankles or knees, joint laxity or functional instability also seems to predispose players to injuries, in particular of the hamstrings, groin, and knee.

Less use of preventive protocols by young players, specifically balance and proprioception exercises, increase the risk of injury, especially passing the higher categories.

The level of competition is also a risk factor because the risk of injury increases with the level of competition from amateurs to elite athletes.

Poor management of training workload leads to a higher risk of injury during matches.

Physical and psychosocial stress appears to increase the injury risk. However, the role of testing the level of stress of the footballers is still generally underestimated.

Close matches (with <4 days) do not allow a complete recovery and lead to early muscle fatigue during matches: influencing decision-making and technical skills, coordinative adjustments are less, increasing the injury risk.

10.1.4 Epidemiology of Injuries

Epidemiological surveys on football injuries have been implemented in Europe since the end of the 1970s, particularly in the northern countries. At that time, these research studies focused on amateur or semi-professional footballers. They described some typical injuries for footballers and the possibility of reducing their incidence. Injury was defined as any physical damage that occurred during football activities (scheduled matches or training sessions) and resulted in the player being unable to participate fully in future training sessions or matches. A player was considered injured until the team doctor allowed full participation in team training and match play. Re-injury was defined as an injury in the same location and of the same type as the player had suffered previously [1].

The review of literature suggests that data of most of the studies are similar [2], with most injuries involving the lower extremity (75.4–93%). Head/spine/trunk injuries occur more often than upper extremity injuries (64–86.8%). The most frequently injured areas in the lower extremity were the ankle (17.0–26%) and knee (17–23%) (Fig. 10.1). In youth players, the area most affected by injury was the lower extremity (61–89%), followed by the head/trunk/spine (9.7–24.8%), and the upper extremity (4.0–24.8%) [3].

The most common types of injuries are contusions, sprains and strains. In the majority of studies, the incidence has been calculated as between 12 and 35 injuries per 1000 h of outdoor games for adult male players and 1.5 and 7.6 injuries per 1000 h of training. In indoor players, the inci-

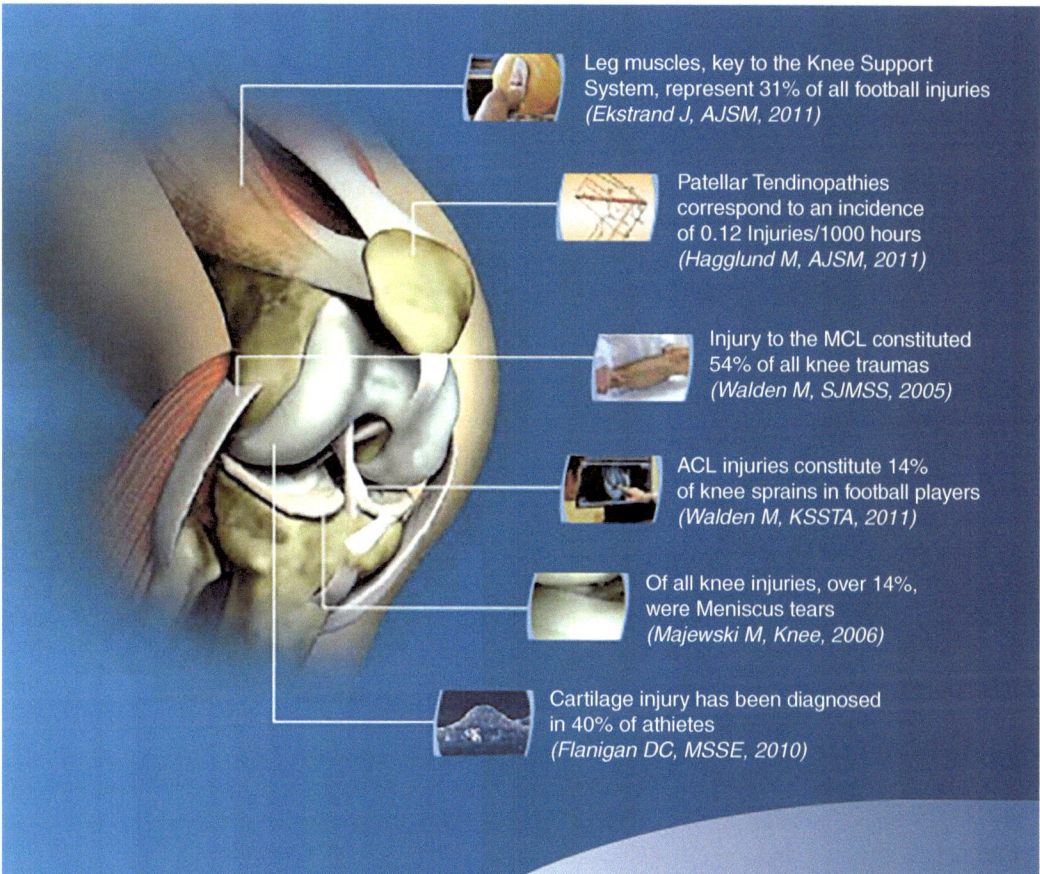

Fig. 10.1 More important knee injuries in football

dence of injury seems to be higher. Muscle injuries, especially to the hamstrings, are the most common in modern football. Joint/ligament sprains, predominantly to the ankle and knee, are also frequent, and may result in long lay-off from training and matches. Although children playing football have fewer injuries than adults, with up to 70% of injuries being mild in nature, the number and severity of children injuries in football are increasing.

The UEFA Champions League represents the highest expression of club level football in the world. Since 2001, UEFA has implemented an injury survey among Champions League clubs, with the aim of reducing injuries that, at this level, have a high economic impact. Prof Jan Ekstrand [3], one of the pioneers of football injury epidemiology, leads the group study for this project. The UEFA Champions League (UCL) Injury Study involves 25 top level European football clubs from 10 different countries and regular data with information on the football activity exposure and injuries situation of each player are collected and sent to the group study. The goals of this project are to establish an injury profile, collect information about rehabilitation and return to sports, and implement specific prevention programs. These studies became very important to identify common injuries at that level of football as well as their characteristics.

In the past 20 years, training and match volume has notably increased due to competition interests, media pressure, economic issues, and global enhancement in professionalism of football, as an important economic domain. However, according to the UEFA injury study, the global risk of injury has not increased because the improvement of preventive and rehabilitative protocols is counterbalancing the progressive increase in intensity of matches, except for muscle injuries, namely hamstrings injury.

The injuries incidence changes greatly depending on the level of play, the workload during training, and the frequency of matches. Injury control is possible due to the improvement of athlete healthcare, metabolic and energetic control, and to the implementation of programs of prevention, including correct management of athlete's loads with player's rotation in official matches.

According to the UCL injury study, a professional football team can expect approximately 50 injuries that cause time-loss from play each season, which equates to two injuries per player per season. The impact of injuries on team performance can therefore be considerable because, on average, 12% of the squad is unavailable due to injury at any point during the season [4]. In modern football, this means a notable economic impact with some teams reportedly losing millions of Euros due to injury with the probability of losing important players and yielding negative results in competitions. These considerations justify an adequate investment in medical care, including devices and professional staff.

Most injuries occur during a match where there is a five times higher risk of injury compared with training. Data from The UEFA Champions League show that the risk of injury remained constant in the past decade. During a match, data show that injury incidence increases during the last part of each half. There is also evidence that overuse injuries have a higher incidence during the preseason, while there are different trends of seasonality linked to different regions and their specific environmental conditions.

The most common injury in football (Fig. 10.2) is thigh strain, typically affecting the hamstring muscle group. Thigh strain represents approximately 17–22% of all injuries and a typical 25-player squad can expect ten thigh strains each season, with seven hamstring and three quadriceps strains.

In general, muscle injuries represent 20–37% of all time-loss injuries in men's professional football, 18–23% in amateurs, and 92% of all injuries affect the four big muscle groups in the lower limbs. Hamstrings injury are the most frequent muscle injury in elite soccer players (37%); it can lead to 80 days loss in a season, re-injuries are frequent and very often occur within 2 months. Furthermore, muscle injuries occur more frequently and with greater severity on the dominant leg. The knee is also a typical location in football injuries, with ACL being the most concerning, and mediatic, injury despite relatively low incidence (<1% of all injuries); statistics show that 94% of players return after 10 months to training, but only 65% after 3 years still play at the same level. The hip and groin are another common injury location with difficulties regarding diagnosis, treatment approach, prevention, and return to play criteria. According to Werner (UEFA injury study, 2009), [4] a team will have seven groin injuries each year with a lay-off time of more than 4 weeks. Finally, ankle injuries account for 10–18% of all injuries in elite players. In football, around 50–81% of ankle injuries are sprains. More recent reports show a decrease of approximately 50% of ankle injuries, and this may be due to prevention strategies, including neuromuscular training, taping, better surfaces, and referee sanctions.

Foul play covers 14–37% of total injuries in football, in 35–80% of cases there appear to be an injury from contact between two players.

The number of re-injuries has recently become a hot topic, leading to the rehabilitation methodology discussion regarding time-based or functional progression in return to sports

Women's football has gained more and more importance in the past few years. The number of participants is rapidly increasing together

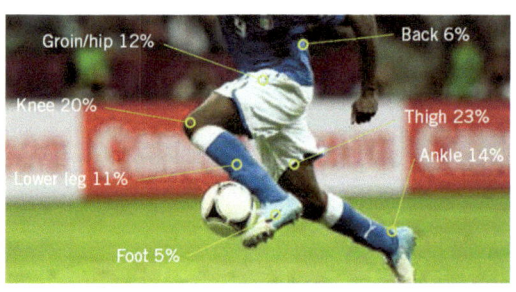

Fig. 10.2 Most important locations of football injuries

with professionalism. According to the most recent FIFA data, there are approximately 40 million women footballers in the world. Injury patterns are largely similar, but females suffer relatively more knee injuries and men suffer more groin injuries. Female players have a two to three times higher risk of ACL injury compared with their male counterparts. Females also tend to sustain their ACL injury at a younger age and have a higher risk of injury, especially during match play, whereas no relevant gender-related difference seems to exist during training.

10.1.5 European Championship Data

The results from the first years of the study suggest that although normally the professional clubs have effective strategies to avoid overloading their players, the intense match schedule for many top players towards the end of the season might have some negative effects on these players' performance and health, namely in final season European and World Cups.

The 2002 World Cup in Korea/Japan had an increased risk of injury, and players/teams often under-performed in that tournament. These findings were later repeated at EURO 2004 in Portugal and, since then, in every World and European Cups.

EURO 2004 in Portugal, 45 injuries occurred (39 in matches and 6 during training).

EURO 2008 in Austria—Switzerland, 56 injuries occurred (46 in matches and 10 during training).

EURO 2012 in Poland—Ukraine, 28 injuries occurred (19 in matches and 9 during training) (Fig. 10.3).

During EURO 2004, the thigh was the most common injury location (22%) followed by the ankle (17%), lower leg (14%), and hip/groin (14%). Sprains (ligament injury) were the most dominant injury type at EURO 2008 ($n = 16$, 29%), and nine of these injuries were to the ankle and seven to the knee. The 15 muscle strain injuries mainly occurred in the thigh ($n = 6$), calf ($n = 4$), and groin ($n = 2$).

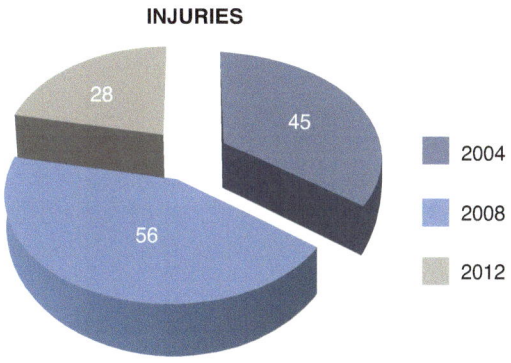

INJURIES

2004
2008
2012

Fig. 10.3 Number of injuries in 3 European Cups

If we compare the total of injuries from Euro 2004 to Euro 2012, the number and severity of injuries tends to decrease in National Teams and became closer, or even better than, UEFA Champions League results (UCL) (Fig. 10.4).

10.1.6 Rehabilitation and Return to Play

Clarifying what "return to sport" means is fundamental because the term allows for various interpretations. Not all studies agree on a single meaning, and the definition of functional recovery remains debated. A standardized, medically supervised on field rehabilitation program for football players based on measurable criteria instead of time frames can provide the basis for a complete functional recovery and return to team competition.

The FIFA (Federation Internationale de Football Association) has proposed the F-MARC test battery for physical performance in football (soccer) players. These tests provide normative data regarding warm-up, flexibility, soccer skills, power, speed, and endurance for healthy players and mean values for similar age groups and skill levels. The player's profile may also be used by the physician and the physical therapist in monitoring the recovery after an injury. These tests will likely reconcile the main goal of surgeons (to obtain the safest return to sports for their patients) with the main goal of coaches (to obtain the fastest return to competition for their players).

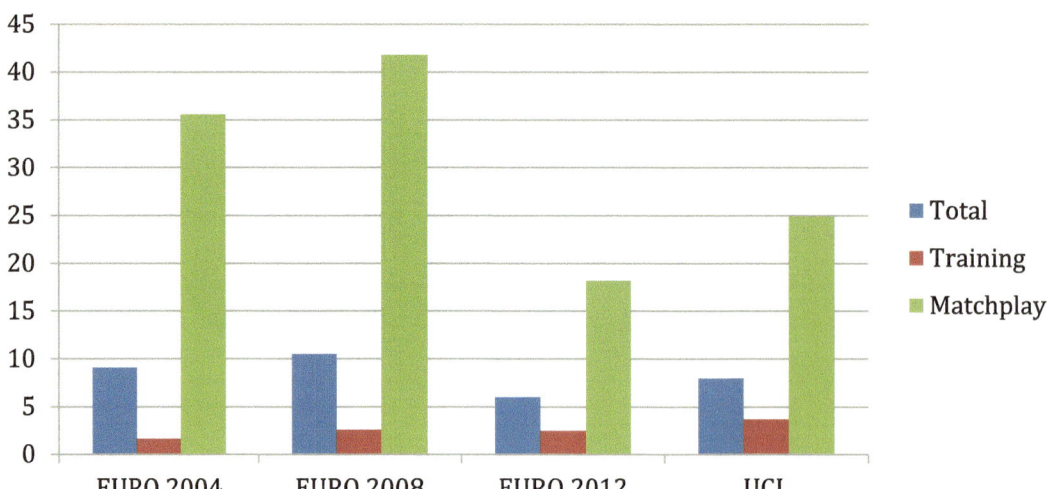

Fig. 10.4 Injury incidence in 2 European Cups and UCL comparation

The right time of return to sport and psychological factors, such as the fear of re-injury, play an important role in reconditioning motor patterns.

The risk of re-injury is very high in the subelite categories, as there are not enough funds to have an adequate medical staff.

10.1.7 Preventive Strategies

Soccer-related injuries are associated with both non-modifiable factors, such as sex and age, and modifiable factors, such as those that can be improved through programs that influence force, balance, and flexibility, especially in young age. The general aspects of injury prevention in football includes several aspects: proper preparation and health care, overuse injuries prevention and injuries prevention programs, neuromuscular training, adequate rest and sleep, adequate dietary and energetic supplementation, adequate warm up and cool down, adequate post-match recover strategies, appropriate equipment, safe environment, safe return to play, if possible, and turn over when there are close games to play.

Specific exercises are required to develop strength during stretching to cope with eccentric forces during rapid movements [5].

Nordic hamstring exercise reduces ischiocrural injuries by 50%; however, especially in the amateur categories, not having a supporting medical staff, the preventive and rehabilitative part is not carried out correctly, increasing the risk of re-injury.

The FIFA 11+ injury prevention program [6] was developed in 2006 to address this matter, under the leadership of the FIFA Medical Assessment and Research Centre and in collaboration with the Oslo Sports Trauma Research Center and the Santa Monica Orthopaedic and Sports Medicine Center. The program comprises a complete warm-up procedure aimed at injury prevention in soccer players. It includes 15 structured exercises, is available as printed material or online, and is easily executed. The exercises consist of core stabilization, eccentric thigh muscle training, proprioceptive training, dynamic stabilization, and plyometric exercises, all performed with proper postural alignment.

Program effectiveness was confirmed by various studies involving female and male players that revealed significant decreases in the incidence of non-contact injuries. In 2016, the warm-up program "FIFA 11+ Kids" was launched with the intention of preventing and reducing the number and severity of football-related injuries [7] by enhancing children's fundamental and

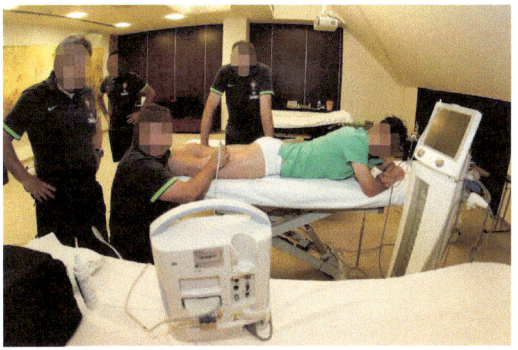

Fig. 10.5 Medical team: sonography regular control of muscle injuries

sport-specific motor skills through a range of evidence-based exercises.

The explanation contemplates factors such as stadium and training camps conditions, adequate rest and fatigue control, better recover strategies, coaches methodology, fair play, referees intervention, better quality of medical support (Fig. 10.5), and effective prevention with more adequate treatments and better criteria in return to sports.

References

1. Fuller CW, Ekstrand J, Junge A, Andersen TE, Bahr R, Dvorak J, et al. Consensus statement on injury definitions and data collection procedures in studies of football (soccer) injuries. Scand J Med Sci Sports. 2006;16:83–92.
2. Ekstrand J, Hägglund M, Waldén M. Injury incidence and injury patterns in professional football: the UEFA injury study. Br J Sports Med. 2011;45:553–8.
3. Waldén M, Hägglund M, Ekstrand J. UEFA Champions League study: a prospective study of injuries in professional football during the 2001–2002 season. Br J Sports Med. 2005;39(8):542–6.
4. Jones A, Jones G, Greig N, et al. Epidemiology of injury in English Professional Football players: a cohort study. Phys Ther Sport. 2019;35:18–22.
5. Rösch D, Hodgson R, Peterson TL, et al. Assessment and evaluation of football performance. Am J Sports Med. 2000;28:S29–39.
6. Sadigursky D, Braid JA, De Lira DNL, Machado BAB, Carneiro RJF, Colavolpe PO. The FIFA 11+ injury prevention program for soccer players: a systematic review. BMC Sports Sci Med Rehabil. 2017;9:18. Published 2017 Nov 28. https://doi.org/10.1186/s13102-017-0083-z.
7. Eirale C, Ekstrand J. Epidemiology of injury in football. Aspetar Sports Med J. 2019;8

Youth Football

Clemens Memmel, Werner Krutsch,
Angelina Lukaszenko, and Oliver Loose

11.1 Characteristics of the Sport

The *"FIFA Big Count"* report of 2006 estimated that there are more than 260 million football players around the world, most of them under 18 years old. The group of young athletes shows the overall greatest increase, with 32% since the year 2000. The popularity of football among children is unparalleled, and the access to club football is much easier compared to other sports. Football as a sport is characterized by simple and well-known match rules and no specific demands for expensive equipment. Furthermore, being a member of a team improves social skills and self-confidence. The positive side-effect of team sports is considered to be highly valuable, espe-

cially during childhood and adolescence. Apart from the pitch, football has its own enormous fan culture with innumerable clubs and celebrities, who also serve as idols for young people. Practically every child has their own role model and their favorite club, which leads to an identification with the sport. These characteristics explain why children and adolescents are so affected by this sport.

11.2 Physiological and Biomechanical Demands on Athletes

In professional football, the main purpose of training sessions in adult ages is to improve the physique and technique of the athletes to meet or even exceed the physiological demands of the sport, such as long-lasting endurance for field players or high response capacity for goal keepers. Deficits in endurance or strength can lead to sporting failure. In comparison, youth football on an amateur level pursues different targets as well. Especially for children up to 11–13 years, having fun during training and matches and creating a supporting environment within the team are at least as important as winning a match.

Nevertheless, the physiological demands of football on young athletes are very similar to those in adult football, although they clearly vary

C. Memmel
Department of Pediatric Surgery and Orthopedics,
Children's University Hospital Regensburg (KUNO),
Campus St. Hedwig, Regensburg, Germany
e-mail: Clemens.Memmel@klinik.uni-regensburg.de

W. Krutsch (✉)
SportDocsFranken in Nürnberg, Nürnberg, Germany
e-mail: Werner.Krutsch@klinik.uni-regensburg.de

A. Lukaszenko
Burjeel Hospital, International Knee and Joint Center,
Abu Dhabi, United Arab Emirates
e-mail: info@knee.ae

O. Loose
Department of Orthopedics, Olgahospital,
Stuttgart, Germany
e-mail: o.loose@klinikum-stuttgart.de

© The Author(s), under exclusive license to Springer-Verlag GmbH, DE, part of Springer Nature 2022
G. L. Canata, H. Jones (eds.), *Epidemiology of Injuries in Sports*,
https://doi.org/10.1007/978-3-662-64532-1_11

in quantity. Football requires physical skills that depend on the position taken in the field. Whereas central defenders might succeed with height and strength, midfielders might need high velocity or a certain sense of reading a game to play their position effectively. The young players have to develop technical abilities and handling with the ball as well as endurance and a stable physical condition to achieve performance during the whole match. Training methods in youth football include physiological adaptation processes such as an increase in muscle volume, progression in proprioception or improvement in endurance, but also represent fun and team-building exercises.

To adapt to the lower physiological demands of the young, football associations implemented specific rules in youth football regarding, for example, the weight and size of the ball or the length of a match. In comparison to adult football, smaller measurements of the field meet the limited endurance of children and the lower strength to pass the ball, and the reduced number of outfield players results in fewer duels involving body contact.

In youth football, it is essential to consider the fact that the body is under constant change and that there are striking differences between prepubescent and pubescent children that subsequently result in different injury patterns. The forces that affect the body during the match are of multiple types, degrees, and directions. They range from indirect shear forces during direction-changes to direct contact forces, e.g., during head-to-head contact in a heading duel. To absorb any kind of kinetic energy and therefore withstand these forces without injury, a sufficient physical condition provided by well-trained muscular stabilizers in combination with a solid bone structure is essential. Therefore, attending training sessions on a regular basis is crucial for meeting the physical demands of football.

11.3 Epidemiology of Injuries

In general, football has a relatively low risk of major injuries in youth ages. There are differences in injury incidence and types of injury between prepubescent and pubescent players due to diverse biomechanical settings of the musculoskeletal system. That is the reason why children aged 7–12 years are unlikely to sustain overuse syndromes or ligament injuries but more often suffer from bone fractures of the long bones.

The injury risk, especially for major injuries, increases with age. The overall injury incidence of pubescent players (age 13–19) ranges from 2–7/1000 h of football exposure and is significantly higher than that of prepubescents. In the 13–19 years age group, 60–90% of injuries are caused by trauma and 10–40% are overuse syndromes. Over all age groups, the most affected body region is the lower leg (60–90%). Minor injuries are mostly found in the ankle, thigh, and foot, whereas the knee is the joint most affected by major injuries. In adults, muscle strains of the thigh are the most common injuries in football. In comparison, children sustain fewer muscle injuries because forces affecting the muscle are transferred to and neutralized in cartilage, ligaments, or bones. This is why the most frequent diagnoses in pubescent players are ligament sprains (30%) and concussions (20%), followed by muscle strains (16%). Concerning the types of overall injuries in pubescent football, contusions are the most frequent, followed by sprains, fractures, and wounds.

Numerous studies have shown that the injury risk is much higher during competition than during practice. Whereas training injury incidence stays nearly constant for athletes aged 13–19 ranging from 1 to 5 injuries per 1000 h of training, competition injury incidence increases during aging (15–20 injuries/1000 h match exposure for athletes >15 years). Especially severe injuries such as fractures or serious ligament strains occur more often during competition due to frequent player–player contacts, which is the most common injury mechanism in pubescent youth football. Non-contact injuries, as the second most common injury type (e.g., supination trauma of the ankle joint), occur more often during practice in relation to match exposure.

Concerning the epidemiology of injuries depending on sex in general, research has shown that female athletes have a significantly higher

Table 11.1 Epidemiologic facts on injuries in children's football

Epidemiology of injuries in children's football
Football is a relatively safe sport with low risk of major injuries
The risk of injury increases during aging
The most affected body part is the lower limb, mainly knee and ankle joints
Injuries occur more often during the game than during practice
Girls have a significantly higher risk of getting injured than boys

injury incidence than male football players. In addition, girls tend to sustain more ligament injuries than boys, such as ACL ruptures, most likely due to hormonal influence, which especially affects the structure of connective tissues such as the ACL (Table 11.1).

11.4   Rehabilitation and Return-to-Play

There are several specifics in youth football compared to adult football that must be considered in injury management. Early and sufficient emergency management of occurred injuries is the fundament for an adequate healing process of football injuries, and in children's football, it is organized differently than in adult football. Because of different anatomic circumstances in junior football players with their growing bones and changes in neuromotorical ability, treatment strategies also show different techniques and goals. These differences include both surgical treatment techniques (e.g., fractures of the growth plate area) and conservative treatment strategies (e.g., time for hospitalization or rest in football after concussion). Although children are capable of faster bone healing and young athletes may need shorter healing periods, it is important to put no pressure on timing to return-to-play. It is crucial to favor a complete healing process and to emphasize full recovery of functionality such as speed or strength because of possible deficits after long time periods. Especially after overuse syndromes in elite youth football, a consequent pausing period has to be discussed with the athlete, parents, and coaches.

11.5   Prevention Strategies

Implementing preventive measures in the daily routine of youth football is the best way of protecting children from football-associated injuries. The key to prevention is the understanding of the different injury mechanisms such as body or non-body contact, which influences risk and protection behavior of young players. In addition to the steps taken by the football organizations as mentioned before, several measures to avoid injuries caused by body contact have already been established such as wearing shin guards during competition or implementing stiffer penalties after elbowing an opponent's head. Improving prevention of non-contact injuries means improving the physical condition of the athletes by performing specific exercises for enhancing proprioception, coordination, and muscular stabilizers. This is why FIFA created an evidence-based preventive warm-up program "FIFA 11+". To meet the special needs of children, FIFA even adjusted the program to generate a special program called "FIFA 11+ for Kids," which is a pre-training and pre-competition warm-up program for children aged 7–13 years that includes seven different playful exercises and training workouts. In a cluster-randomized controlled trial, the program was shown to reduce up to 48% of football-related injuries by enhancing motor performance.

Another prevention strategy is the right adjustment of training intensity to the physical capacity and biomechanical state of the young athletes. Practices have to be conducted at age-appropriate intensities. Over the past decades of junior football, it has become routine to promote talented players into the next higher age group or even to double the match exposure by competing in both age leagues in amateur teams. It is highly recommended to avoid such stresses on young athletes in order to prevent them from overuse syndromes or a higher risk of major injuries that could endanger their physical and even mental health. Simultaneously, the possibility of a higher injury risk should be considered if female athletes play in male football teams on a pubescent age level because of higher practice and competition intensites compared to the ones of female football leagues of the same age group. To date, there is not clear evidence to support restrictions concerning such mixed teams.

By considering the epidemiology of injuries in children's football, understanding the injury mechanisms of the growing body, including its physiological and biomechanical demands, and by implementing preventive strategies into daily routines, coaches, athletes, physiotherapists, and practitioners in sports medicine can keep football a safe sport for children.

11.6   Injury Prevention Assessment

Understanding the mechanism of possible injury can lead to a better treatment or to creation of a proper prevention strategy. As time and research have shown, for example, the mechanism of an anterior crucial ligament rupture usually occurs upon impact during a bad landing after jumps, where knee valgus and big internal rotation of the femur bone are present. Knowing these important facts, assessment and prevention is becoming easier to establish.

We want to present a small assessment plan for a non-adult football player that can be performed on a daily basis to better understand the biomechanics of a young player.

1. Manual joint and muscle assessment: this can help detect restrictions in movements and properly establish a potential treatment plan. Based on this examination, especially young players can return to sport after any injury or simply continue the training or match without injury after all (Fig. 11.1).
2. Video analysis of the movement can lead to a quick and simple functional diagnosis of a young player. Potential dynamic malpositioning that is not easily visible during a match, such as a dynamic valgus during landing or

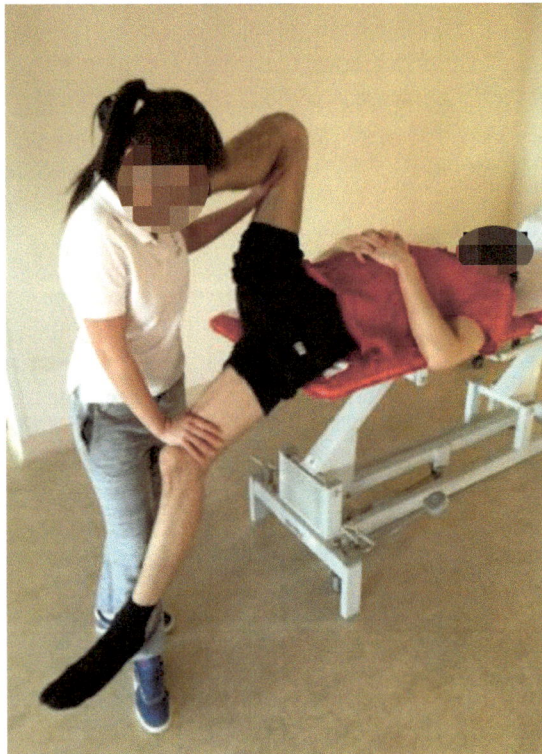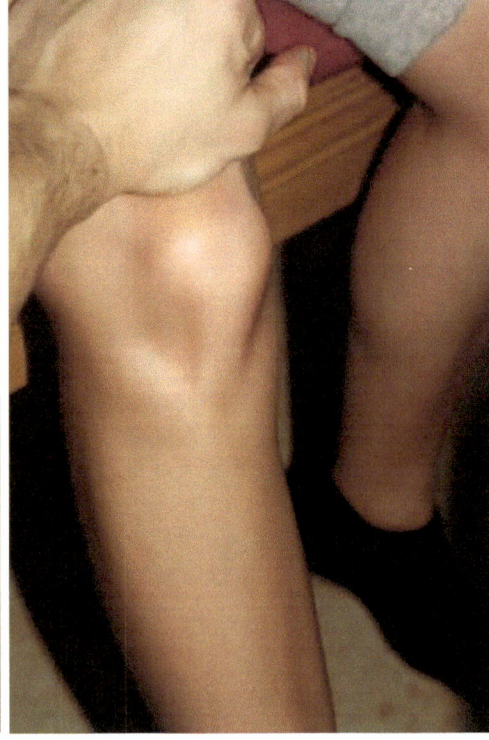

Fig. 11.1 Manual assessment (Courtesy of the Carolina Medical Center Warsaw)

running, can lead to serious injuries. Through video analysis, such risk factors can be detected (Figs. 11.2, 11.3, and 11.4).

3. Muscle torque analysis can be performed on children or adolescent players above 11 years, due to the size of the measuring device. Muscle torque analysis could be done during the process of training to better detect muscle imbalance. That kind of measurement could be additionally supported by an EMG (electromyography) signal.

To be better prepared for any match and training session, especially in different environments, it is crucial to have a prevention assessment plan for young football players.

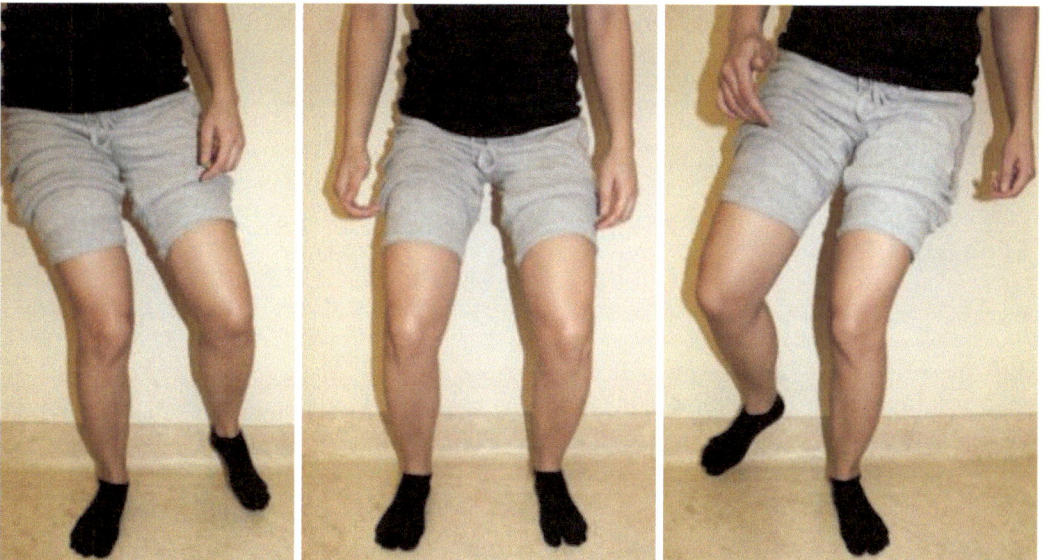

Fig. 11.2 Video analysis of the technique of one- and two-legged jumping and landing (Courtesy of the Carolina Medical Center Warsaw)

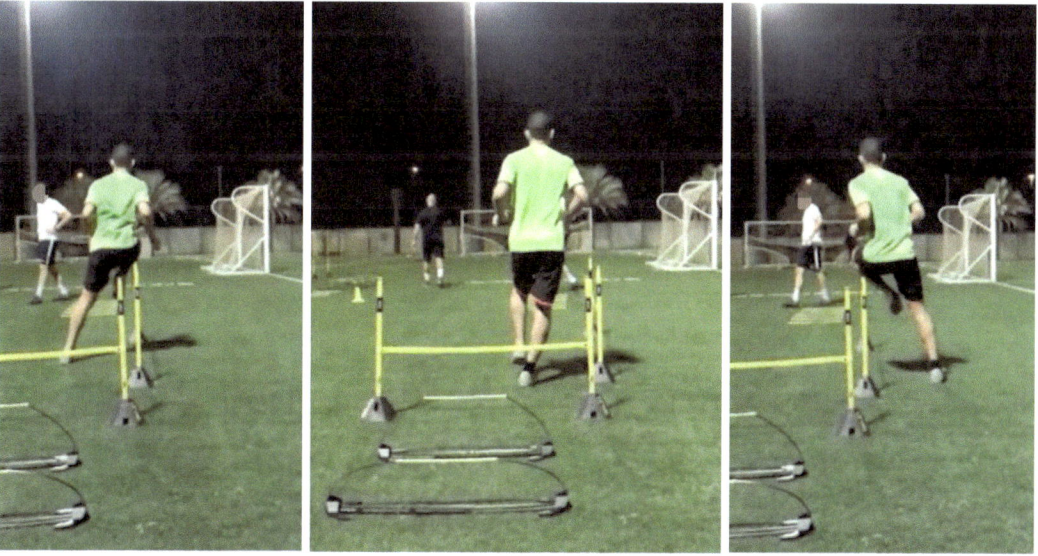

Fig. 11.3 Video analysis of a player on the pitch during a training session (Courtesy of Atomics Football Abu Dhabi)

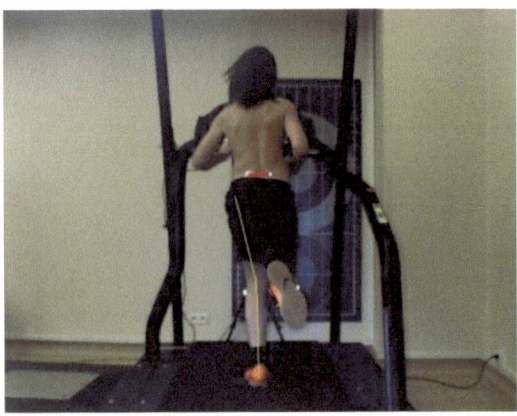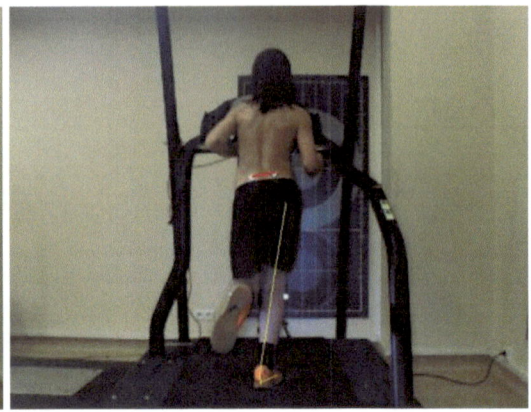

Fig. 11.4 Video analysis of a young football player during running (Courtesy of the Carolina Medical Center Warsaw)

Suggested Reading

Faude O, Rößler R, Junge A. Football injuries in children and adolescent players: are there clues for prevention? Sports Med. 2013;43(9):819–37.

FIFA Communications Division, FIFA Big Count 2006: 265 million playing football, Zurich

Krutsch W, Voss A, Gerling S, Grechenig S, Nerlich M, Angele P. First aid on field management in youth football. Archiv Orthopaedic Trauma Surg. 2014;134(9):1301–9.

Rössler R, Junge A, Bizzini M, Verhagen E, Chomiak J, Fünten K, Meyer T, Dvorak J, Lichtenstein E, Beaudouin F, Faude O. A multinational cluster randomised controlled trial to assess the efficacy of '11+ kids': a warm-up programme to prevent injuries in children's football. Sports Med. 2018;48(6):1493–504.

Rössler R, Junge A, Chomiak J, Němec K, Dvorak J, Lichtenstein E, Faude O. Risk factors for football injuries in young players aged 7 to 12 years. Scand J Med Sci Sports. 2018;28(3):1176–82.

Handball

12

András Tállay, Lior Laver, Kai Fehske,
and Leonard Achenbach

12.1 Characteristics of the Sport

Handball is a worldwide popular Olympic ball sport and one of the most popular ball sports in Europe. Today, handball is played in 199 countries with 19 million players worldwide in over 800,000 teams played year-round at professional level. Combining international competitions with club and national teams, elite players play between 70 and 100 matches a year. While some countries remain stable in regard of members, some countries have risen to over double in just some years, such as Hungary (2011–2017) from 24,000 to 65,243 registered handball athletes (Fig. 12.1).

During the last decades, the game of handball went through several changes (i.e., rules, court, and shoe design) which made it much faster and dynamic. Handball is characterized by intense body contact, frequent intermittent running, demanding one-on-one confrontations, and quick direction changes and cutting movements in combination with challenging technique and coordination elements like catching, throwing, passing, and dribbling. Aggressive contact is an integral part of the game and often used not only to stop the opponent but also to intimidate opponents from approaching the goal. The changes of the game and increased number of players and games played annually have resulted in higher number of traumatic and overuse injuries. The physiologic load that each player is exposed to varies depending on their age, playing level, playing position, and total number of players in the teams [1].

Handball is in the top five sports in terms of number and severity of injuries. Apart from being a throwing sport during which a high number of loads are transferred to the upper extremity in general and more particularly to the shoulder joint, handball is also a contact and pivoting sport. It involves lots of running, turning, and jumping during the game, exposing the joints of the lower extremity to high levels of mechanical stress. Contact-related injuries represent a large fraction of all handball injuries. All these factors predispose handball players to develop osteoarthritic changes of the upper and lower extremity.

A. Tállay (✉)
National Institute for Sports Medicine,
Budapest, Hungary

L. Laver
The Royal Orthopaedic Hospital—NHS Foundation
Trust, Birmingham, UK

K. Fehske
Department of Surgery II, University of Würzburg,
Würzburg, Germany

L. Achenbach
Clinique Générale Annecy, Annecy, France

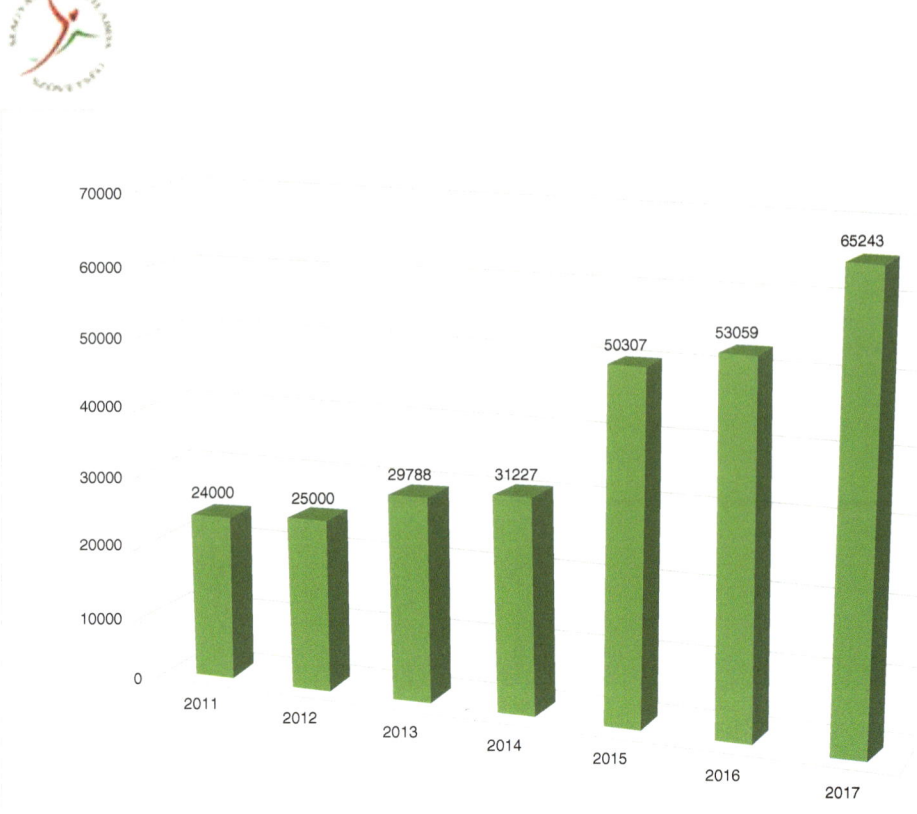

Fig. 12.1 The increase of the number of competitive handball players in Hungary (Bardóczy, Hungarian Handball Federation, Annual Report 2017)

In children and adolescents, the sport is going through a phase of increasing professionalization as well. Handball schools and academies are being created in many countries and international competitions have been implemented in youth players. Fortunately, the benefits of handball on the health and social development of these young athletes exceed its disadvantages. However, a major problem is the large number of young players affected by serious ligament injuries, mainly of the knee joint. Many players suffer from injuries very early in their handball career. In the long term, such severe injuries may lead to early-onset degenerative changes and osteoarthritis (OA) [2].

12.2 Physiological and Biomechanical Demands on Athletes

To become an elite handball player, next to high level of skills, good speed and acceleration, muscle strength and endurance, power, agility, flexibility, balance and coordination, reaction time, and cardiovascular endurance are required. Besides the physical parameters' mental abilities, like analytic and tactical ability, motivation and self-confidence and coping with pressure situations are determining as well. To set up an optimal body composition and stamina for a handball player we have to follow the evidence-based age- and sex-based formulas to avoid the undesired medical overuse conditions [3]. The training of handball players should target the ability to perform specific high-intensity actions throughout the game and to rapidly recover during the less intense periods. To evaluate the effectiveness of the training methods periodical physiological and biomechanical screening is recommended. Throughout the annual training program elite players typically practice once or twice a day, and in competition phase they play 1–2 games/week.

The mean height of players varies among different nations and can range for males from 178 ± 4 cm to 194 ± 2.1 cm and in females from 164 ± 4.3 cm to 178 ± 3.4 cm. Information on physical characteristics of players playing different positions can help coaches match the training program to the specific attributes of players who play similar positions. To date, taller players have better chances to play on the highest level. Mean body mass ranged from 77 ± 7.5 kg to 107 ± 7.9 cm in male players. In females there is also a wide range detected in body mass from 60 to 72 kg [3].

Motion analysis has shown that depending on the playing time and playing position handball players cover a distance of up to 6.5 km per game; therefore aerobic capacity is needed as they are constantly running up and down the court during the games. In addition, high levels of anaerobic power allow the players to achieve explosive acceleration or power when it is needed. This potential may be needed in numerous situations in handball such as when athletes sprint to receive the ball, then recover quickly, and sprint again with many repetitions occurring in a single match. Unfortunately only a limited published data exists on the on-court physiological demands of the handball players, but it appears that especially the explosive capacity decreases in the last 10–15 min. The activity pattern of the different playing positions' players varies on a wide range [3].

The study by Póvoas et al. aimed to analyze elite handball players' physical and physiological demands during match conditions. Different locomotor categories were defined: standing still, walking, jogging, fast running, sprinting, backwards movement, sideways medium-intensity movement, and sideways high-intensity movement and playing actions studied were jumps, shots, stops when preceded by high-intensity activities, changes of direction, and one-on-one situations. They found that during the games average distances covered were 4370 ± 702.0 m. Around 80% of the playing total time was spent standing still (43.0 ± 9.27%) and walking (35.0 ± 6.94%), and only 0.4 ± 0.31% accounted for sprinting. Effective mean HR was 157 ± 18.0 bpm (82 ± 9.3% of HRmax) and total HR was 139 ± 31.9 bpm (72 ± 16.7% of Hrmax). Most intense periods of the game were higher during the first half than during the second half ($p \leq 0.05$). Handball is an intermittent exercise that primarily utilizes aerobic metabolism, interspersed by high-intensity actions that greatly tax anaerobic metabolism. Additionally, exercise intensity decreases from the first to the second half of the match, suggesting that neuromuscular fatigue may occur during the game [4].

Wagner et al. have tested specific physical performance in male team handball players and the relationship to general tests in team sports. It was demonstrated that general and handball-specific performances are separate components. Recommendations to strength and conditioning professionals and coaches in handball were presented.

To conclude, handball is a physically demanding complex game for both sexes. Playing handball includes powerful upper body movements such as maximal ball throwing and tackles of opponents as well as forceful lower limb muscle actions during vertical jumping, sideways and backwards running, rapid sprinting, and directional changes during fast breaks during the entire match. The physical training of different positions' players should be organized in a more individualized manner in the future according to specific requirements in defense and offense. Considerable sex-specific variations in the physical demands exist in handball. Physical training of female handball players may potentially benefit from a greater focus on aerobic training elements. Conversely, male elite players would seem to benefit from an increased training focus on anaerobic exercise elements and strength training. Additionally, the physical demands differ greatly between various playing positions both in offence and defense, reflecting almost similar trends in both male and female elite players.

To find the optimal biomechanical and exercise physiological screening program is still controversial. Several laboratory- and game-specific telemetrical instruments are available, but the effectiveness and cost benefit are still controversial [5].

Some nations have implemented a mandatory screening program for their (elite) handball athletes. One example from Hungary is as follows (Figs. 12.2, 12.3, and 12.4):

The possible positive fitness effects of handball for recreational players were studied as well.

The participation in regular recreational handball training was associated with positive cardiovascular, skeletal, and muscular adaptations, including increased maximal oxygen uptake, increased muscle enzymatic activity, and improved bone mineralization as well as lower fat percentage. These findings suggest that playing handball on recreational level may be an effective health-promoting activity for young adult men [6].

Body composition
Age: 31 years Weight: 59.00 kg Body fat: 8.10 kg Skeletal muscle: 28.50 kg Arm ballance: 0.10 kg Arm dominance: Right Leg ballance : 0.10 kg Leg dominance: Right
Height: 174 cm Body water: 37.30 kg Fat free mass: 54.22 kg Body mass index: 19.49 kg/m2
Waisthip ratio: 0.83

Circulatory system: Endurance absolute: 45 bpm Endurance actual: 60 bpm Autonom ballance: 100.00 % Adaptation inde x: 84.00 ms
Respiratory system: Vital capacity: 112.00 % Forced vital capacity: 111.00 %
Metabolic Hemolytic Mechanic Metabolysm: Ph: 7.41 cHCO3: 23.40 mmol/l cBase: 0.90 mmol/l cK: 4.20 mmol/l cNa: 136.00 mmol/l cCa: 1.13 mmol/l
Lactate: 0.70 mmol /l Hemoglobin: 14.90 g/dl Hematocrit: 44.00 % Glucose: 5.70 mmol/l Creativ cinase: 63.00 u/l
Static: Foot ballance: 4.00 % Ballance dominance: Right Foot rotation: 0.00 ° Rotation dominance: , Push up ballance: 4.00 % Push up dominance: Left Push up muscle ballance: 0.00 % Push up muscle dominance: , Spine scolozis: Poor, Spine posture: Good Spine mobility: Poor Spine portural: Poor Spinal: Normal
Endurance: Move form: Trademill running(km/h) Relative aerob capacity max: 48.50 O2ml/kg/min Oxygen pulse max: 15.92 O2 ml Aerob threshold power: 10 Wv.Km/h Anaerob threshold power: 14 Wv.Km/h Maximum performance: 16 Wv.Km/h Training relief: 11.90 mmol/l Training relief: 118 bpm

Neuromuscle coordination: Power bilateral pull performance: 0.00 W/Kg Power bilateral push performance: 5.41 W/Kg Weight: 59.00 Kg Bilateral arm push: 412.00 N Relative explosive strength pull: 0.00 % Relative explosive strength push: 71.18 % Bilateral push power: 319.00 W Jump test left leg performance: 17.32 W/kg Jump test right leg perfo rmance: 14.68 W/kg Juming test leg diference: 0.26 % Jump test bilateral leg performance: 22.75 W/kg Jumping test bilateral: 22.75 W/Kg Bilateral jump: 863.00 N Bilateral jump relative : 149.10 %
Nervous system: Execution speed: 4366.00 mHz Focusing: 88.30 % Sensorimotor function: 95.00 % Decision making skill: 48.00 % Visual vigilance: 58.00 % Error: 6.00 %

Fig. 12.2 Mandatory screening program for an elite Hungarian elite handball player

OSEI
SPORTKÓRHÁZ

Hungarian National Institute of Sports Medicine
Dr. Ágnes Soós, general director
Performance Diagnostics Department
Dr. Péter Kovács PhD head of department
1123 Budapest, Alkotás u. 48.
EMail: kovacspeter@osei.hu
Phone: +36 30 299 7286

Training zones

Movement form	Treadmill running(km/h)
MmaxHR:	179 bpm
Mmax speed/performance:	16
MmaxLactate:	9.0000 mmol/l

Intensity zone	Movement form	Time p:pm	Speed/Power km/h/W	Sys hgmm	Dias hgmm	Hr bpm	Hr rest bpm	Hr dif bpm	Lactate mmol/l	Rlavg msec	Vo2Max ml/kg/p	O2HR ml
nyugalom		00:00	0	94	62	64	64	0	0.7000	286		
aerob extenzív		02:00	8			123	113	10	0.6000			
aerob intenzív		04:00	10			140	135	5	1.8000			
aerob intenzív		06:00	12			154	151	3	2.6000			
anaerob extenzív		08:00	14			170	163	7	5.8000	510		
anaerob intenzív		10:00	16			179	150	29	9.0000	392	48.5000	15.9200
megnyugvás		14:00	5	121	64	118	118	0	11.9000			

Fig. 12.3 Exercise physiology: treadmill test methodology for elite handball players

12.3 Epidemiology of Injuries

Handball injuries are diverse in terms of the mechanism of injury, how they present in individuals, and how the injury should be managed. Although the rules of handball try to make it fair and safe, acute and overuse injuries are very common. The risk of injury is significantly higher during matches than during training; most probably the reason is higher speed and intensity during matches, and more contact with opponent players. According to basic epidemiological studies the knee and ankle injuries are the most common sites for acute injuries, with the ankle being more common in most studies; however the most sever acute injuries involve the knee (i.e., ligamentous injuries). The knee, shoulder, and lower leg are common sites for overuse injuries [3].

Epidemiological data on handball-specific injuries have been generated either through retro- and prospective cohort studies or from observational studies during international tournaments. The used term for "sport injury" is problematic and not consistent; therefore to compare the data of different studies is difficult [5]. There are many ways to classify sports injuries based on the time taken for the tissues to become injured, tissue type affected, severity of the injury, and which injury the individual presents with. Depending on the classification the severity and prevalence of handball injuries vary.

Some data have been generated from federation or insurance-related injury registries and from specific injuries such as the anterior cruciate ligament (ACL) reconstruction registries. Aman et al. reported on large number and incidences of injuries as well as injuries leading to permanent medical impairment (PMI) from the Swedish national injury database [7]. Giroto et al. investigated the incidence and risk factors for handball injuries in 21 handball teams participating in the two main Brazilian championships during a season ($n = 339$ elite Brazilian handball players). Three hundred and twelve injuries were reported in 201 athletes. The injury incidence rate during training and matches reached 3.7/1000 h and 20.3/1000 matches, respectively. Ankle (19.4%) and knee (13.5%) were the body regions most affected by traumatic injuries; shoulders (44.0%) and knee (26.7%) were the body regions most affected by overuse injuries. This study showed that athletes with previous injury have a high risk of developing an overuse injury [5].

Tatrai et al. compared their Hungarian injury register data to those from the German. According to the regulation of the national federation, all first league male and female teams have to use a compulsory injury register. The results of the 2017/2018 season show that the most vulnerable joints are knee and ankle in accordance with the international data. The frequency of injuries was 15% higher than that in Germany (98

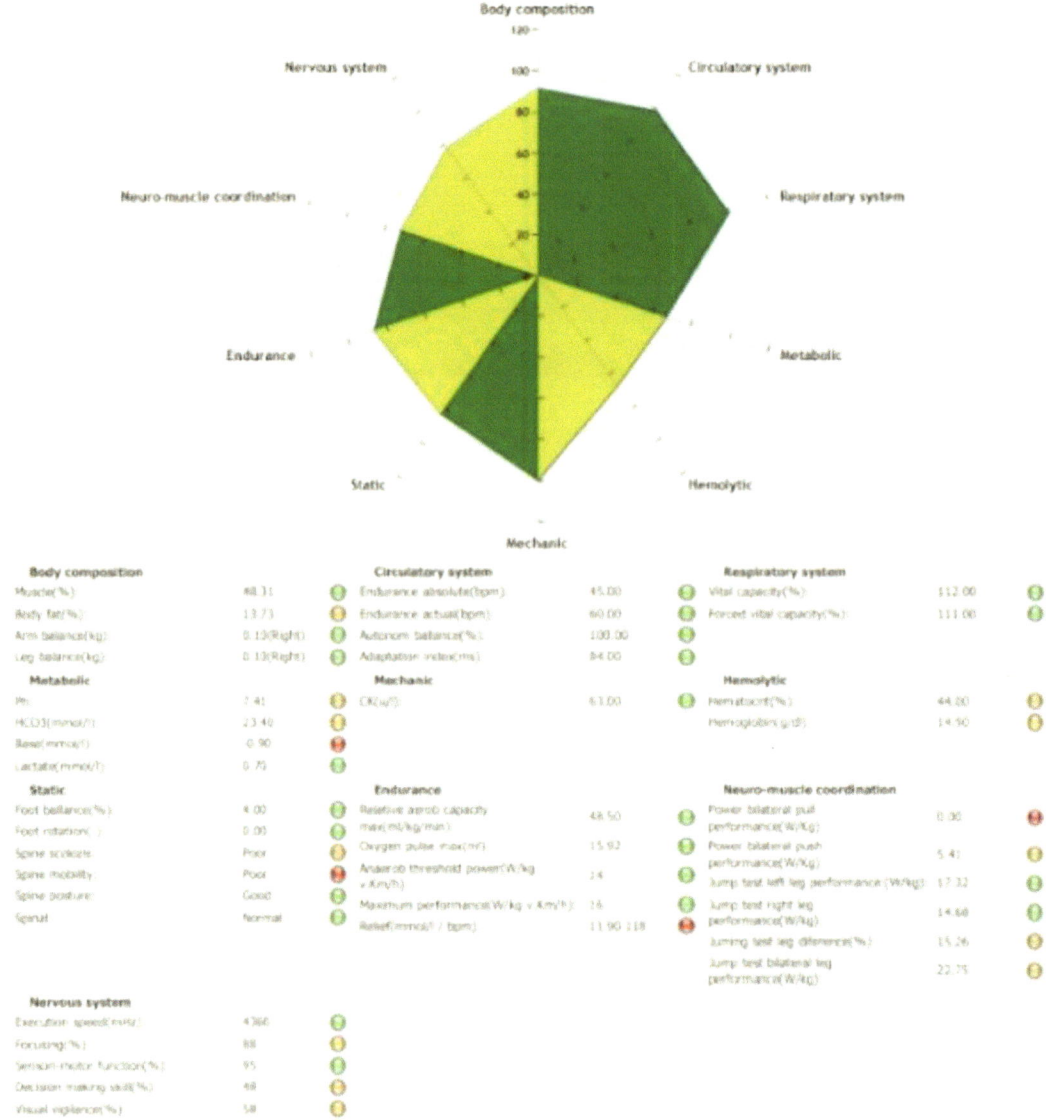

Fig. 12.4 The medical report to the green color deviation from the optimal range, the yellow color with slightly suboptimal, and the red color represents a significant depar-ture. The colorful web shows the average values seen until the last page of the rating which is determined by the colors of the worst modular indicator

injury/1000 h vs. 78 injuries/1000 h). The injury prevalence per player for 1000 playing hours was 2.8. The weakness of the Hungarian injury register is that it focuses only on the game injuries, providing no data from the training session. German registry data found that 54% of all injuries occur during training circumstances.

Nielsen et al. reported the injury incidence of 221 players in one season with 4.6 per 1000 playing hours and 11.4 per 1000 match hours. The upper extremity was involved in 41% of the injuries including 21% finger sprains. Ankle sprains were the most common injury (33%), and overuse injuries accounted for 18%. The risk of reinjury was 32%. Contact mechanism was 31% of all injuries. Forty percent of the injuries were minor injuries, treated by the players themselves. 73% of the players were absent from handball for more than 1 week, and 41% of the players had complaints 6 months after the end of the season.

This study shows that injuries in handball are serious and cause long-term consequences for the players. In most of the injuries both intrinsic and extrinsic factors were involved, and prophylactic intervention in these cases demands changes in more fields [1]. *Mónaco et al.* studied the influence of position, category, and maturity status on the incidence and pattern of injury in handball players, across two seasons. The 164 players were categorized into youth (133) and adults (31), and per position: 27 goalkeepers, 67 backs, and 70 wings and pivots. Injury incidence in youth was 6.0 per 1000 total hours [CI 95%, 4.8–7.2] (14.9 match [9.7–20.1] and 3.7 training hours [2.7–4.6]; $n = 142$ injuries), and in adults 6.5 per 1000 total hours [4.4–8.6] (22.2 match [8.8–35.6] and 3.0 training hours [1.3–4.6]; $n = 48$ injuries). There were significant differences in knee ($P = 0.01$) and cartilage injury ($P = 0.05$) according to the playing position. There were significant differences according to age category in ankle ($P = 0.03$), head ($P = 0.01$), thigh ($P = 0.05$), muscular injury ($P = 0.02$), and apophysitis ($P = 0.04$) for biological maturity state. Adult handball players had more ankle and muscle injuries than youths. Pivot and wings (second line) had more knee and cartilage problems. A higher incidence of apophysitis was found in immature youth players [7]. Lindblad et al. registered 570 handball injuries prospectively in a well-defined geographic area of 124,321 inhabitants. The incidence of handball injuries was 46 per 10,000 inhabitants per year, and the ratio was twice as much in women (61 per 10,000 per year) than men (31 per 10,000 per year). Nearly two-thirds of the injuries were ligament sprains and tears, and 12% were fractures. Sixty-eight percent of the injured players were not able to return to handball within 1 week. Surprisingly, 8% of the minor injuries resulted in a sick leave of more than 6 days [8].

12.4 Rehabilitation and Return to Play (RTP)

Once an injury occurred, one of the most burning questions from the player and coaching staff is regarding "when can they return to play."

Management of a safe RTP is a challenging task and varies from injury to injury. Returning too soon can increase your risk of reinjury or developing a chronic problem that will lead to a longer recovery. Waiting too long, however, can lead to unnecessary *deconditioning* and it can also influence the results of the team.

The rehabilitation strategies are constantly improving. The basis for a safe RTP and adequate rehabilitation is a fast and correct diagnosis. Once the team physician sets up the diagnosis, the healing process is led by the physiotherapists, addressing the normal tissue biologic and biomechanic requirements for healing, gradual restoration of muscle strength deficits, and building towards handball-specific training, with or without contact initially, when appropriate, before full RTP [2].

Addressing the player's conditioning status during the rehabilitation process is important in facilitating a timely and safe RTP. The team physician can determine the best time for returning to play. Basically, two main principles exist, the time based or criteria based. All strategies are aim for being pain-free, no swelling, full range of motion, and full or close to full (90%) strength. It is important to keep in mind that even when all criteria are present, biology—like graft healing after ACL reconstruction—still plays a crucial role. It is extremely important to take extra care with the injured part for several months. The time-based return to sport limit for the most frequent serios knee injury—ACL—has increased by 50% in the last few years, from a minimum of 6–9 months. RTP for different injuries and different body sites varies on a wide spectrum. Most handball injuries have evidence-based RTP protocols. Compromises to decrease the minimum RTP time are sometimes required with elite players at the most important (AC, WC, Olympics) tournaments, during intense competition; however, it should be avoided in other scenarios.

12.5 Prevention Strategies

Injury prevention in handball has been shown to be successful over the years, with handball being one of the sports leading the way in this field. It is one of the only sports where such strategies have been shown to be effective for both lower limb injuries and shoulder injuries. The knowledge and understanding regarding prevention of especially acute lower extremity injuries in handball have improved substantially in the last two decades. More is known about injury mechanisms, who is injured, and, most importantly, how these injuries can be prevented. The risk of sustaining an acute lower extremity injury, including ACL injuries, has been shown to be reduced by 50% through implementing injury prevention exercise programs (IPEPs) as structured warm-up program on a regular basis in handball [9].

Overuse injuries in handball are also a well-known problem, and recent work has shown that it is possible to reduce the risk of shoulder overuse injuries in handball by 28% by performing a set of exercises during the warm-up [9].

The elements of injury prevention in handball aim to address identified risk factors for injuries in the sport as well as high-risk situations and mechanisms, through improving elements of coordination, strengthening, stabilization, and proprioception, contributing to performance enhancement as well as injury prevention. Structured warm-up programs including neuromuscular training, agility, balance, strength, and playing technique exercises, designed to improve knee and ankle control during landing and pivoting movements, have been shown to reduce ACL injuries and proven to be an efficient way of implementing such strategies. Success highly depends on the compliance of players.

It is recommended to have regular preseason screenings to detect potential risk factors for injuries, e.g., cardiovascular problems, muscular imbalances, and athletic and neuromuscular deficits. Moreover, performance diagnostics that identify the athletes' individual needs for improvement can assist in increasing physical condition and general performance and thus contribute to reducing acute and chronic injuries.

It is recommended to have all national associations to include an injury prevention module in their trainer education curriculums and to designate an official staff member as "safety promotion ambassador" of the federation. And last but not least, all sustained injuries should be reported to trainers and coaches and should be systematically recorded at club and national level, in order to identify individual and situational risk factors, to monitor injury trends, and to evaluate the effects of the measures taken [10].

References

1. Nielsen AB, Yde J. An epidemiologic and traumatologic study of injuries in handball. Int J Sports Med. 1988;9(5):341–4.
2. https://www.verywellfit.com/when-is-it-safe-to-return-to-sports-after-an-injury-3119404
3. Laver L, Landreau P, Seil R, Popovic N, editors. Handball sports medicine basic science, injury management and return to sport. Springer Berlin, Heidelberg; 2018.
4. https://www.researchgate.net/publication/221726733_Physical_and_Physiological_Demands_of_Elite_Team_Handball
5. Wagner H, Sperl B, Bell JW, von Duvillard SP. Testing specific physical performance in male team handball players and the relationship to general tests in team sports. J Strength Cond Res. 2019;33(4):1056–64. https://doi.org/10.1519/JSC.0000000000003026.
6. Hornstrup T, Løwenstein FT, Larsen MA, Helge EW, Póvoas S, Helge JW, Nielsen JJ, Fristrup B, Andersen JL, Gliemann L, Nybo L, Krustrup P. Cardiovascular, muscular, and skeletal adaptations to recreational team handball training: a randomized controlled trial with young adult untrained men. Eur J Appl Physiol. 2019;119(2):561–73.
7. Mónaco M, Rincón JAG, Ronsano BJM, Whiteley R, Sanz-Lopez F, Rodas G. Injury incidence and injury patterns by category, player position, and maturation in elite male handball elite players. Biol Sport. 2019;36(1):67–74. https://doi.org/10.5114/biolsport.2018.78908. Epub 2018 Oct 15
8. Lindblad BE, Høy K, Terkelsen CJ. Handball injuries: an epidemiologic and socioeconomic study. Am J Sports Med. 1992;20(4):441–4. https://doi.org/10.1177/036354659202000413.
9. Myklebust G, Engebretsen L, Braekken IH, Skjølberg A, Olsen OE, Bahr R. Prevention of noncontact anterior cruciate ligament injuries in elite and adolescent female team handball athletes. Instr Course Lect. 2007;56:407–18.
10. http://cms.eurohandball.com/PortalData/1/Resources/1_ehf_main/3_download_pdf/Safety_in_Sports_-_Fact_sheet.pdf

13 Ice Hockey

Kazumi Goto and Jacques Menetrey

13.1 Characteristics of the Sport

Ice hockey is a popular winter sport in many countries and consist of pushing and hitting a small rubber puck into a goal with a hockey stick. The game is played between two teams of six players, including one goalkeeper and five ‘field’ players. The playing time is three periods of 20 min each. Players perform between 10 to 20 min of a 60-min game. Each shift lasts approximately 30–40 s and is very intense. Time of recovery between shifts may vary from 45 s to a few minutes. The game requires high skating skill, an excellent physical conditioning, outstanding technical capabilities, eyes–hands coordination, and good capacity of trunk–lower limbs dissociation. Although the rules are slightly different between categories such as gender and age, one of the sport’s major characteristic is the intense body contact called body checking allowed in the men’s category. Body checking can occur in the middle of the ice, against the boards, at high speed, with and without the presence of a disputed puck (Fig. 13.1).

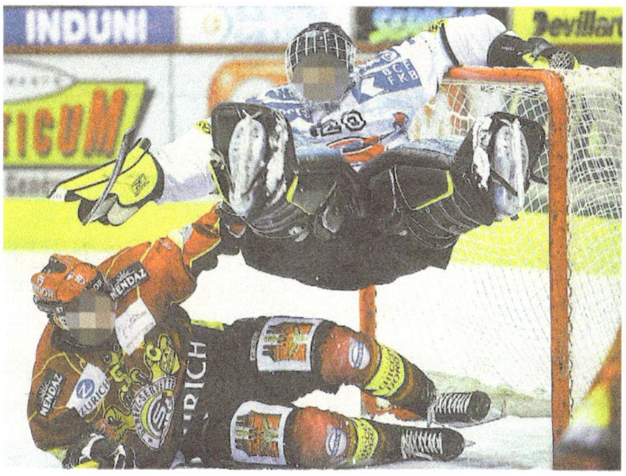

Fig. 13.1 Contact in ice hockey can occur anytime and should be practiced, anticipated when possible, and performed respecting the rules

13.2 Physiological and Biomechanical Demands on Athletes

Because of the above characteristics, ice hockey players require high anaerobic characteristics and a good aerobic basis. Since this sport includes frequent body contact and high intensity intermittent skating, it requires strength and volume

K. Goto (✉)
Center for Sports Medicine and Exercise, Swiss Olympic Medical Center, Hirslanden Clinique la Colline, Geneva, Switzerland
e-mail: kazumi@kgorthop.com

J. Menetrey
Center for Sports Medicine and Exercise, Swiss Olympic Medical Center, Hirslanden Clinique la Colline, Geneva, Switzerland

Orthopaedic Surgery Service, University Hospital of Geneva, Geneva, Switzerland
e-mail: Jacques.Menetrey@hirslanden.ch

G. L. Canata, H. Jones (eds.), *Epidemiology of Injuries in Sports*,
https://doi.org/10.1007/978-3-662-64532-1_13

of the upper body as well as a robust lower body. There are significant differences in VO2 during skating. As already mentioned, both the aerobic and anaerobic energy systems are important during a game. The peak heart rates during a shift is over 90% of max-heart rate (Max-HR) and the average rate when a player is on the ice is approximately 85% of Max-HR. By the nature of the game (repetitive boost of energy), a wide range of muscle fibre composition can be found amongst ice hockey players. One study looked at the muscle fibre composition in 25 college and professional players, and showed that slow twitch fibre composition of the vastus lateralis ranged from 20 to 71%. There was no difference in the percentage of type I fibres between positions (goalkeepers 47.4%, defensemen 51.7% and forwards 48.1%).

There are little data on the flexibility of hockey players. The results of trunk flexion, trunk extension and shoulder extension for professional hockey players showed similar scores between forwards and defensemen. Goalkeepers showed significantly better flexibility for hamstring, trunk flexion and shoulder extension. Compared to other sports (basketball, baseball, football player, shotput and discus throwers, swimmer, and wrestler), hockey players exceeded the other athletes (except swimmers) on wrist, hip, knee and ankle flexibility.

13.3   Epidemiology of Injuries

Ice hockey is associated with many risk factors for injuries, such as intentional and unintentional collisions, high velocity, sudden changes in direction and traumatic hit by the stick or the puck or against the boards. Consequently, a wide variety of injuries occur, but contusions are the most frequently encountered. Epidemiological studies from the NHL have reported that facial injuries and concussions were frequent. During the Olympics, ice hockey was the sport with the highest risk of injury, affecting 13–35% of hockey players [1].

Based on the study of 1685 hockey players from all NHL teams [2], competing through the 2006–2007 to the 2011–2012 seasons, the overall regular season incidence density was 15.6 injuries/1000 player hours and 0.7 illnesses/1000 player hours. Based on the recorded time on ice, the injury rates were roughly threefold higher at 49.4 injuries/1000 player hours and 2.4 illnesses/1000 player hours. In this study, the most commonly injured body regions were the head (17%), thigh (14%) and knee (13%). In another study about NHL players, injury involved the head and face in 40%, the lower body in 31%, the upper body in 22% and the spine or trunk in 8%.

This study [2] also described risk factors by position. Compared with the forwards, the defensemen were more likely to report a game-related time-loss injury. There was no difference between defensemen and goalkeepers or forwards and goalkeepers. Injuries were significantly more frequent in the first period (49%) than in the second (26%) and the third (25%) periods. Game-related injuries and illnesses were also unequally distributed over the course of a season. Specifically, injuries trend towards an increase at the summer camp and early season to peak in October/November and increase again nearing the end of the regular season [2].

Facial (including dental) and head injuries were the most commonly injured body parts. In men's World Championship, facial injuries comprised 72% of head injuries [3], amongst them most were laceration caused by the stick. Injury rate for dental injuries was 0.5 (9.5%) and for eye injuries 0.1 (1.4%)/1000 player-games.

The upper extremity is a common site for ice hockey-related injuries and accounts for the highest percentage (44%) for youth ice hockey injuries according to one study. Players aged 12–17 years had the highest rate of upper extremity injuries (47% of all reported injuries) which was twice that of all other age groups. The shoulder was the most common location for an upper body injury (50%) and the rate was 1.5/1000 player-games. Acromioclavicular (AC) joint sprain (51%) and glenohumeral joint injury (40%) were the most frequent diagnostic. The fingers (14%), wrist (11%) and hand (11%) injuries were in second, third and fourth place in upper body injuries, respectively [3]. However, injuries of hands account for a high number of days lost.

Lower-body injuries account for 30% to 45% of all hockey player-related injuries [4]. The knee was the most common part with 47% of the lower body injuries. Medial collateral ligament (MCL) sprain was the most common knee injury (56%), and most of them were grade I injuries (51%). Anterior cruciate ligament (ACL) ruptures represented 11% of all knee injuries associated with meniscus tears in 15% of cases. Ankle and thigh injuries in NHL players account for the second and third most common lower body injuries. In addition, femoroacetabular impingement (FAI) is one of the known specific pathologies in goalkeepers due to the unique style (the butterfly technique), especially in higher level.

Concussions account for approximately 13% of all sports-related injuries. Ice hockey is the second highest rate of all sports-related concussion, with 1.2–1.6 per 1000 player game-hours. Concussions occurred more frequently in games (2.5/1000) compared to practices (1.2/1000). The most common cause for concussion was a check to the head (52%). Younger players are more likely to be concussed; this may be due to the lack of experience in body checking, in the control of their emotions and in the management of the game. Players tend to be more skilled in proper checking technique at an older age. In a previous report, 33–43% of impacts causing concussion were the result of illegal contact. The 'centre' position had the highest risk of concussion (25–31%), then 15–20% of concussion concern the defenseman and 17–19% the wing position. The majority of concussions occurred during the first period (42–47%) [4] (Tables 13.1 and 13.2).

13.4 Rehabilitation and Return to Play

There are various protocols of treatment and rehabilitation depending upon the type of injury. This section focused on the major injuries encountered in ice hockey.

Table 13.1 Ice hockey injuries by anatomic region [2, 3]

Diagnosis	2007–2013 Men's world champion ship games	2006–2012 All NHL teams 376 games
Total number	**528**	**5184**
Face	129 (24%)	–
Knee	76 (14%)	13%
Shoulder + clavicle	59 (11%)	12%
Head	58 (11%)	17%
Fingers + thumb + hand	31 (6%)	7%
Ankle + lower leg	25 (5%)	8%
Groin + hip + pelvis	23 (4%)	9%
Teeth	20 (4%)	–
Thigh	22 (4%)	14%
Chest + throat	19 (4%)	4%
Foot + toes	16 (3%)	6%
Neck + upper back + lower back	16 (3%)	3–7%
Wrist	13 (2%)	2%

Table 13.2 Mechanism of injury reported during regular season and postseason games between 2009 and 2012 (NHL) [2]

Mechanism	Injury frequency (%)
Total	**1877**
Body check	536 (28.6%)
Received	451 (24.0%)
Delivered	85 (4.5%)
Non-contact	277 (14.8%)
Incidental contact	268 (14.3%)
Hit by puck	253 (13.5%)
Shot	236 (12.6%)
Pass	17 (0.9%)
Contact with environment	176 (9.4%)
Other intentional player contact	139 (7.4%)
Fighting	68 (3.6%)
Unknown	160 (8.5%)

Recovery time and criteria for return to play for the AC joint injuries is different between the grades of injury (from I to III). As a first step for returning to play (RTP), the player should have full recovery of strength and range of motion on the affected side. Thus, the recovery time is variable. RTP after a lesion of grade 1 can be considered at 2–3 weeks, while a lesion of grade III takes 6 weeks. The use of tape and AC joint pads can protect the AC joint and reduce the pre-emptive pain by decreasing contact forces.

When properly rehabilitated, the period for return to play after a grade I MCL injury is of 0–2 weeks, 2–4 weeks for a grade II injury and 6 to 8 weeks for an isolated MCL grade III injury, although those are often surgically fixed to prevent residual laxity. In rehabilitation, recovery of ROM and quadriceps strength and neuromuscular capacities are crucial, as for other knee injuries.

When it comes to rehabilitation after the treatment of FAI, 3–4 months is needed to participate in skating/hockey drills. This functional programme is divided into a four-phase rehabilitation protocol, of which the phases are athlete dependent. Therefore, an individual athlete's rehabilitation agenda should be taken into consideration.

A few protocols specific to ice hockey players after ACL reconstruction have been reported [5]. A four-phase criteria of ice skating was proposed: early, intermediate, late and return-to-sport. The early on-ice phase (>16 weeks) gradually exposes the athlete to the specific skating requirements. The intermediate on-ice phase (>20 weeks) aims to develop power and initiate anticipated changes of direction. The late on-ice phase (>6 months) aims to develop anaerobic endurance and initiate unanticipated changes of direction without contact. Finally, the return-to-sport phase (>9 months) can allow non-contact and contact drills, scrimmages and games.

Most low ankle sprains are managed non-operatively with a functional rehabilitation programme because the ice hockey boot provides excellent support and protection for low ankle sprains. Return to play is usually allowed within a few days to a week after a minor sprain, while more severe injuries may require from 6 to 8 weeks for a complete ligament healing. Syndesmotic injuries are the ones that may require the longest period to heal.

Concussion is one of the most severe injuries in ice hockey. The 2012 Zurich Consensus Guidelines stated that a concussed athlete should not return to play in the same game. If a concussion is confirmed, the player should be immediately removed from the game or practice. An athlete should never be allowed to return to a game or practice on the same day. The athlete should be consulted with a follow-up by a doctor who is familiar with the treatment of concussions and should be withheld from all physical exercise until they are asymptomatic at rest. Once the athlete reports the baseline, the athlete can resume the stepwise protocol (6 steps) under the supervision of the doctor or athletic trainer. Then, they can gradually increase activity and participation for training.

13.5   Prevention Strategies

Several injury prevention strategies have been reported over the years with mixed results. The use of full-face masks, visors, helmets and mouth guards have significantly reduced the incidence of eye, dental and facial injuries. However, there is no evidence that helmets can protect against concussion, and although debated, mouth guard seems to have limited effect in reducing the severity of a concussion. Flexible boards have allowed for a significant diminution in concussion and shoulder injuries. A study about neck and spinal cord injuries in hockey showed that one of the major causes of injury was pushing or checking a player from behind into the boards. As a result, Hockey Canada decided to impose a major penalty for checking from behind in the 1985–1986 season. Since the implementation of this rule and of educational programmes increasing the awareness about the danger of checking from behind, the annual incidence of spinal cord injury has decreased, but has not been eliminated. However, it raises the importance of a prevention campaign aiming at the respect of the game's rules. Therefore, because the overall number of head and neck injuries in ice hockey remains very high, additional interventions are necessary. Concussion must be prevented at all levels of the game. A recent article reviewed the effectiveness of the video 'Smart Hockey: More Safety, More Fun' on knowledge prevalence about the dangers of concussion. The study reported an immediate improvement in concussion awareness, but the effect was lost after 2 months. Prevention of concussion includes a good physical conditioning, flexible boards, a perfect focus when the player is on the ice, the respect of the rules and of his partners and opponents. Referees/officials are in charge of the safety of the game, and as such, they play a central role in the prevention of concussion and more generally of severe injuries. Finally, the governing body of ice hockey should not only enforce the present rules, but should think of modifying some of them to better protect the players and their heads.

References

1. Laprade RF, Surowiec RK, Sochanska AN, et al. Epidemiology, identification, treatment and return to play of musculoskeletal-based ice hockey injuries. Br J Sports Med. 2014;48(1):4–10.
2. McKay CD, Tufts RJ, Shaffer B, Meeuwisse WH. The epidemiology of professional ice hockey injuries: a prospective report of six NHL seasons. Br J Sports Med. 2014;48(1):57–62.
3. Tuominen M, Stuart MJ, Aubry M, Kannus P, Parkkari J. Injuries in men's international ice hockey: a 7-year study of the international ice hockey federation adult world championship tournaments and Olympic winter games. Br J Sports Med. 2015;49(1):30–6.
4. Mosenthal W, Kim M, Holzshu R, Hanypsiak B, Athiviraham A. Common ice hockey injuries and treatment: A current concepts review. Curr Sports Med Rep. 2017;16(5):357–62.
5. Capin JJ, Behrns W, Thatcher K, Arundale A, Smith AH, Snyder-Mackler L. On-Ice Return-to-Hockey Progression After Anterior Cruciate Ligament Reconstruction. J Orthop Sports Phys Ther. 2017;47(5):324–33.

Olympics

14

Mitchell I. Kennedy, Torbjørn Soligard,
Kathrin Steffen, Gilbert Moatshe,
and Lars Engebretsen

14.1 Introduction

Although high-level sporting competitions of Olympic athletes have been shown to be beneficial regarding reduced risk of disease and increased life expectancy relative to the general population [1–5], it is also related to increased risk of developing musculoskeletal disorders [6–9] resultant of the injuries sustained from years of training and competition. The responsibility of Olympic orthopedic physicians is to protect athletes' health, through prevention, treatment, and rehabilitation of injuries with the assessment of the health status of athletes and their risk of future injury [10]. To aid in establishing these protocols, injury surveillance dur-ing the Olympic Games plays an important role. Surveillance of these events promotes injury prevention by enabling identification of common or severe injuries [11, 12], in addition to characterization of risk factors and mechanisms of injury [13], which is ultimately utilized for the model of Translating Research into Injury Prevention Practice (TRIPP) [14].

14.2 Injury Surveillance in the Olympic Games

In order to evaluate athletes' health and risk of injury with greater specificity, injury surveillance studies have been implemented since the 2008

M. I. Kennedy
Medical and Scientific Department, International Olympic Committee, Lausanne, Switzerland

T. Soligard
Medical and Scientific Department, International Olympic Committee, Lausanne, Switzerland

Faculty of Kinesiology, Sport Injury Prevention Research Centre, University of Calgary, Calgary, AB, Canada
e-mail: torbjorn.soligard@olympic.org

K. Steffen
Department of Sports Medicine, Oslo Sports Trauma Research Center, Norwegian School of Sport Sciences, Oslo, Norway
e-mail: kathrin.steffen@nih.no

G. Moatshe
Department of Sports Medicine, Oslo Sports Trauma Research Center, Norwegian School of Sport Sciences, Oslo, Norway

Department of Orthopedics, Oslo University Hospital, Oslo, Norway

L. Engebretsen (✉)
Medical and Scientific Department, International Olympic Committee, Lausanne, Switzerland

Department of Sports Medicine, Oslo Sports Trauma Research Center, Norwegian School of Sport Sciences, Oslo, Norway

Department of Orthopedics, Oslo University Hospital, Oslo, Norway
e-mail: lars.engebretsen@medisin.uio.no

Beijing Summer Olympic Games [12]. Since implementation, injury surveillance has been routinely performed at all the Olympic Games and findings have been reported in several studies [10–12, 15–18]. Injuries and illnesses were classified as either new (excluding preexisting injuries or injuries not completely rehabilitated) or recurring (athletes that have returned to full participation in former conditions) and included musculoskeletal complaints, concussions, and other medical conditions receiving medical attention throughout the period of the Olympic Games during either competition or training [17]. These studies have provided vital epidemiological data while enhancing injury prevention by stratifying injuries within each respective sport that occurs in both the Winter and Summer Olympic Games. By tracking the occurrence of injuries within each sport, risk factors and mechanisms of injury can be identified, leading to the establishment of preventative measures to reduce the risk of injury [19]. Ultimately, the aim of injury surveillance and TRIPP is not to eradicate injuries from the Olympics, but rather to reduce the rate at which they occur while maintaining the integrity of the sport [16].

The International Olympic Committee (IOC) places high precedence for each National Olympic Committee (NOC) and International Federation (IF) to protect the health of their athletes and actively focus on injury prevention [10]. This is a difficult task, as approximately 1101 injuries occurred within a population of 11,274 athletes competing in the 2016 Summer Olympic Games in Rio de Janeiro [17], and 376 injuries occurred in 2914 athletes competing in the 2018 Winter Olympic Games in Pyeongchang [16]; thus, incidences of injury per 100 athletes over a 17-day span were 9.8 and 12.6, respectively. Though the overall injury rate throughout recurrences of the Summer and Winter Olympic Games has remained fairly constant with at least one injury sustained by 8% [17] to 12% [16, 18] of all athletes [11, 12, 15], changes of sports-specific injury rates have been observed amongst successive Olympic Games. In addition, new sports are introduced to the Games, e.g., skateboarding, speed climbing, and surfing to the

coming Games in Tokyo, which challenges the work on prevention and treatment prior to and during the Games.

The injury rate in a sport may experience incidental deviations as a result of factors like environmental conditions, but they are also susceptible to contents of the Olympic Games program, venue/course designs, and degree of injury awareness amongst athletes and medical staff [11, 12, 15–18]. Awareness begins with understanding injury trends that occur within the population of athletes in successive years, with the most frequent injuries in recent years being sprain/ligament ruptures, bone contusions, and muscle contusions [16, 17]. Sports-specific injury awareness is also vital, as it is reliant on identifiable risk factors and injury mechanisms that can be associated with the components of each sport. This is evident in sports involving high speed, aerial maneuvering, or contact between athletes or with course obstacles, in which a higher proportion of the acute injuries occur within both the Winter and Summer Olympic Games [19], as opposed to overuse or chronic injuries. Furthermore, the setting of injury, being either in training or competition, is also regularly correlated with specific sporting events across both Olympic Games.

14.3 Periodic Health Evaluations

Some conditions are not always accompanied by overt symptoms: therefore, periodic health evaluations (PHEs) are utilized to screen injuries early and implement intervention and management to athletes at risk of injury [20]. Screening by PHE is most commonly utilized in the off-season to provide medical clearance for sports participation, but it is also beneficial in identifying medical conditions that may have been previously overlooked, as athletes occasionally fail to seek medical attention even after symptoms are present [20]. From the data of the injury surveillance studies, sports are frequently identified with distinct injury patterns, with high prevalence of acute injuries in team or high-speed sports, and overuse injuries in technical sports or from repetitive motions. Therefore, the injuries most commonly associated within each sport, identified from surveillance studies, guide physicians in developing sports-specific PHEs that display greater sensitivity in assessing athlete health. An additional aspect of PHEs is identifying deficits resultant of prior injuries. Certain injury types have higher potential for recurrence following injury, which could compromise joint function and stability, or potentially disturb the integrity of neighboring structures [20].

14.4 Translating Research into Injury Prevention Practice

Integration of research into injury prevention is a complex process that must account for the incidence of injuries specific per sport while also taking into account factors that may influence these injuries or the means for treatment. The following is a six-stage framework model proposed by Finch [14], which accounts for not only the risk factors that influence the injuries but also the influences of sports safety behaviors that may affect injury rates. The first stage is that of injury surveillance, assessing injury incidence across both spatial and temporal trends, in addition to quantifying the relative risk of injury across sporting events. Stage two attempts to understand the etiology of the injuries by elucidating the mechanisms of injury through biomechanical models or associating factors with injury cause and severity through epidemiological studies. Identifying potential solutions and preventative measures occurs in stage three, by developing countermeasures to risk factors associated in stage two. Stage four evaluates the formulated preventative measures in "ideal conditions," which contributes to the efficacy of preventative interventions; however, these measures are not without limitations because the nature of the environment of influences and resources within these studies differ significantly from real-world applications. Stage five involves assessment of the available resources for infrastructure and equipment in determining how likely the developed interventions can be implemented into the real-world context of injury prevention from factors of on-field behavior and perception of the risk of injury. Lastly, stage six involves implementing the intervention in real-world context and evaluating its effectiveness; this primarily involves utilization of the stage four interventions while accounting for stage five sports-specific safety cues.

14.5 Future Directions

The role of team physicians can be challenging because of the demands pertaining to high performance, results, and financial incentives. It is also clear that most medical schools and residency programs do not put much emphasis on injury prevention, but rather on the tertiary care involving treatment of injuries and secondary prevention. Improved knowledge on anatomy, biomechanics, and function has led to improvements in surgical treatment of musculoskeletal injuries; however, time loss from injury and the rate of return to play are not ideal. Therefore, it is imperative to focus on injury prevention when taking care of athletes.

Surveillance studies are vital to improve sports-specific injury awareness by physicians in tracking the incidence of severe or moderate injuries, but minor injuries or overuse injuries are frequently overlooked. This may be the resultant of athletes failing to seek medical attention due to the injury severity not being significant enough to fully inhibit sports participation, even though they endure function restrictions or lesser performance. Improving awareness of these injuries especially leading up to Olympic Games is important, to prevent injuries from progressing into more severe conditions that could significantly reduce performance or even completely prevent participation.

Injury awareness improves with each Olympic Games surveillance, but accountability of injury reporting still requires greater attention. Variability of injury reporting is consistently evident between NOCs and Olympic personnel, with both medical personnel groups possessing a significantly small portion of identical injury reports [16–18]. A recent transition to an electronic data collection system has allowed for more feasible entry of injuries by each NOC [16], which facilitates greater identification of risk factors and mechanisms of injury by specificity of sport by providing a collective location for injury reporting across all NOCs. This system also provides a simplified means for reviewing athlete injury history during Olympic events, optimizing patient-specific assessments of injury risk, and supporting physician decision-making in the management of injuries and the ensuing approval for continued competition.

A prevalent theme across the Olympic Games is the inverse relationship that has been consistently identified between NOC size and incidence of injuries within that NOC. A substantial disparity is present in the availability of resources between NOCs [16, 17], with larger delegations usually having well-developed sports medicine communities that allow for a more comprehensive treatment availability for athletes of these NOCs. This ultimately presents an issue of nonuniform health care for athletes across various sized NOCs competing within Olympic Games [17].

14.6 Conclusion

Treating athletes throughout each Olympic Games proves to be a challenging task as each event contains a wide variety of sports competitions in addition to dealing with a changed environment upon successive Games. To support orthopedic physicians in managing injuries across all sporting events, surveillance studies have been implemented to identify the incidence of injuries and risk factors specific to the respective sport of the athlete. This improvement in sports-specific injury awareness not only enables physicians to possess greater preparedness for the occurrence of injuries relative to treatment and performance expectations, but it also enables tailoring of sports-specific injury prevention measures to ultimately reduce the occurrence of these injuries and create optimal safety measures for competing athletes.

References

1. Clarke PM, Walter SJ, Hayen A, Mallon WJ, Heijmans J, Studdert DM. Survival of the fittest: retrospective cohort study of the longevity of Olympic medallists in the modern era. BMJ. 2012;345:e8308.
2. Kujala UM, Sarna S, Kaprio J, Koskenvuo M. Hospital care in later life among former world-class Finnish athletes. JAMA. 1996;276(3):216–20.
3. Sarna S, Sahi T, Koskenvuo M, Kaprio J. Increased life expectancy of world class male athletes. Med Sci Sports Exerc. 1993;25(2):237–44.
4. Teramoto M, Bungum TJ. Mortality and longevity of elite athletes. J Sci Med Sport. 2010;13(4):410–6.
5. Zwiers R, Zantvoord FW, Engelaer FM, van Bodegom D, van der Ouderaa FJ, Westendorp RG. Mortality in former Olympic athletes: retrospective cohort analysis. BMJ. 2012;345:e7456.
6. Drawer S, Fuller CW. Propensity for osteoarthritis and lower limb joint pain in retired professional soccer players. Br J Sports Med. 2001;35(6):402–8.
7. Drawer S, Fuller CW. Evaluating the level of injury in English professional football using a risk based assessment process. Br J Sports Med. 2002;36(6):446–51.
8. Lohmander LS, Ostenberg A, Englund M, Roos H. High prevalence of knee osteoarthritis, pain, and functional limitations in female soccer players twelve years after anterior cruciate ligament injury. Arthritis Rheum. 2004;50(10):3145–52.
9. von Porat A, Roos EM, Roos H. High prevalence of osteoarthritis 14 years after an anterior cruciate ligament tear in male soccer players: a study of radiographic and patient relevant outcomes. Ann Rheum Dis. 2004;63(3):269–73.
10. Junge A, Engebretsen L, Alonso JM, et al. Injury surveillance in multi-sport events: the International Olympic Committee approach. Br J Sports Med. 2008;42(6):413–21.
11. Engebretsen L, Steffen K, Alonso JM, et al. Sports injuries and illnesses during the Winter Olympic Games 2010. Br J Sports Med. 2010;44(11):772–80.
12. Junge A, Engebretsen L, Mountjoy ML, et al. Sports injuries during the Summer Olympic Games 2008. Am J Sports Med. 2009;37(11):2165–72.
13. van Mechelen W, Hlobil H, Kemper HC. Incidence, severity, aetiology and prevention of sports injuries. A review of concepts. Sports Med. 1992;14(2):82–99.
14. Finch C. A new framework for research leading to sports injury prevention. J Sci Med Sport. 2006;9(1–2):3–9. discussion 10
15. Engebretsen L, Soligard T, Steffen K, et al. Sports injuries and illnesses during the London Summer Olympic Games 2012. Br J Sports Med. 2013;47(7):407–14.
16. Soligard T, Palmer D, Steffen K, et al. Sports injury and illness incidence in the PyeongChang 2018 Olympic Winter Games: a prospective study of 2914 athletes from 92 countries. Br J Sports Med. 2019;53(17):1085–92.

17. Soligard T, Steffen K, Palmer D, et al. Sports injury and illness incidence in the Rio de Janeiro 2016 Olympic Summer Games: a prospective study of 11,274 athletes from 207 countries. Br J Sports Med. 2017;51(17):1265–71.

18. Soligard T, Steffen K, Palmer-Green D, et al. Sports injuries and illnesses in the Sochi 2014 Olympic Winter Games. Br J Sports Med. 2015;49(7):441–7.

19. Steffen K, Soligard T, Engebretsen L. Health protection of the Olympic athlete. Br J Sports Med. 2012;46(7):466–70.

20. Ljungqvist A, Jenoure P, Engebretsen L, et al. The International Olympic Committee (IOC) Consensus Statement on periodic health evaluation of elite athletes March 2009. Br J Sports Med. 2009;43(9):631–43.

Formula 1 World Championship

15

Fredrick Fernando, Alessandro Biffi, Fabrizio Borra,
Filippo De Carli, Giuseppe Monetti,
and Felice Sirico

15.1 Introduction

The Formula 1 World Championship is the main and most popular single-seat race competition. Together with Rally, Endurance and Rally Cross, F1 World Championship is organized worldwide according to the FIA (Federation Internationale de l'Automobile) regulations. FIA not only regulates World Championships, such as the Formula 1 World Championship, but also manages a large number of continental championships (i.e. European Rally Championship) and special championships (i.e. historical competition), up to regulating karting and each competition including an automobile.

In these competitions, engineers develop cars with special characteristics and with high performance technologies, including mechanical, electronic, aerodynamic and others. It is not rare that some of these technologies are applied in the automotive industry to improve performance and safety. Although engineers are fundamental in planning and designing these vehicles, the human factor represents a key element. Indeed, an exceptional motor control, sustained cognitive functions, integrity of musculoskeletal system, attentional skills and top level reaction times are required to drive these cars.

Drivers are able to 'push' these vehicles towards their limits to complete a predefined number of laps in a specific circuit in the shortest possible time. These activities expose drivers to several risks, mainly related to possible crashes with other cars or with circuit barriers and to possible overuse injuries in some body systems, such as the musculoskeletal system. Although the driver is usually considered the main actor in the Formula 1 World Championship, it is necessary to underline that the assembly of the vehicle is carried out by mechanics, under the directions of the engineers. The vehicle 'anatomy' is very difficult and requires considerable time and effort to be assembled. Moreover, several adjustments are done during competition preparation stages. Therefore, the assembly of the car also requires a high-demand human involvement. Owing to this concept,

F. Fernando (✉) · A. Biffi
Med-Ex, Medicine & Exercise—Medical Partner
Scuderia Ferrari, Rome, Italy
e-mail: fred@med-ex.it

F. Borra · F. De Carli · G. Monetti
Dipartimento di Diagnostica per Immagini, Ospedale
Privato Accreditato Nigrisoli, Bologna, Italy

F. Sirico
Med-Ex, Medicine & Exercise—Medical Partner
Scuderia Ferrari, Rome, Italy

Sport Medicine Division, Department of Public
Health, University of Naples "Federico II",
Naples, Italy

G. L. Canata, H. Jones (eds.), *Epidemiology of Injuries in Sports*,
https://doi.org/10.1007/978-3-662-64532-1_15

mechanics are subjected to repetitive micro-traumas that can interfere with the integrity of structures in their musculoskeletal system. This scenario explains why prevention of injuries is a key concept in the Formula 1 World Championship from several points of views and it is not only limited to crashes prevention during competition or to drivers' safety.

15.2 Characteristics of Formula 1 World Championship

The Formula 1 World Championship's calendar includes different races in several continents. Each year the list of countries hosting races could be modified according to FIA's agreements. Several international teams participate in the competition, each with two cars and with two official drivers. During the past years, 10 teams took part in the competition with a total of 20 cars. Each team develops a new car for each season, according to FIA technical regulations. Usually, some tests are performed in February, to complete car configuration. The first race is in March and the last at the end of November, covering a 9-month period of races, with two-weeks resting period in August. The total number of competitions per year varies between 20 and 22, with a mean of 2–3 races per month. Some races are designed in a back-to-back way, with two races planned during two consecutives Sundays. Team members reach the site of the race one week before the date of the race itself, usually. Each race lasts almost 2 hours and covers a total distance of approximately 305 kilometres. Therefore, according to the length of the track, each race has a different number of laps to go. Before the official race, usually performed on Sunday, two sections of free practice are planned during Friday (1.5 + 1.5 h) and one section of free practice plus qualification are carried out on Saturday (1 + 1 h). The previous days are used to assemble box and cars, with a mean working time of almost 10–12 hours per day.

15.3 Physiological and Biomechanical Demands of Drivers and Team Members in Formula 1 World Championship

Drivers have to sustain a high-demand task for a long period of time, in a restricted and non-modifiable environment: the cockpit. Actually, Formula 1 cars are able to go beyond the 300 kpm (kilometres per hour) on the straight. Each turn is crossed as fast as possible, usually. Tyres grip, aerodynamic down-force, centrifugal force, track surface imperfections, banked corners and several other factors are determinant in the production of vertical, lateral and longitudinal forces able to interact with drivers' body. As a consequence, the drivers have to 'react' to these forces that could reach three to six times the G-force (gravity acceleration). To perform this control efficiently, drivers have to control their posture and movements through sustained tonic contractions of large muscular groups.

Moreover, vibration in the cockpit, temperature within the cockpit, continuous verbal interaction with team members via radio, visual perception through helmet, and 'fighting' with other drivers, add some other complexity to this system. Other factors act on driver's health and performance. For example, jet lag should be taken into account due to the worldwide distribution of the races. Some races are performed during the evening (i.e. Bahrain Grand Prix, Singapore Grand Prix and others). In some races, the air temperature is a relevant factor (i.e. Singapore Grand Prix) and could affect drivers' performance. Also, difference in food and nutrition could play a part as variable on the drivers' performance. Beyond drivers, each team includes almost a hundred members involved in specific tasks: logistical organization, hospitality activities for guests, restaurants and technical members. Among technical operational members of the team, engineers are involved in car development, design and operational supervision. On the other hand, mechanics are involved in car assembly according to engineers' operational guidelines. The assembly of the car is a complex process, and it is performed several times during each race, forcing engineers and mechanics to sustain prolonged working hours.

These procedures require a high cognitive and attentional demand and have a significant impact on several body systems such as the musculoskeletal system. Indeed, forced and repetitive movements could determine overuse injuries in several structures such as tendons, ligaments and joints structures.

Owing to car architecture, mechanics are forced to maintain prolonged uncomfortable postures able to apply further stressful forces on the musculoskeletal system. If overuse pathologies are the main problem during preparation for the race, acute musculoskeletal diseases could be recorded during the event among mechanics too. Indeed, mechanics are involved in a high-speed, high-intensity procedure: the pit-stop. During the pit-stop, a series of harmonic mechanical procedures are performed on the car, such as tyres substitution, aerodynamic regulations and others. These activities have to be performed as fast as possible and are usually concluded in a few seconds (from 2 to 5 s). During car elevation, tyres mobilization and tyres substitution, mechanics use large muscles groups. These procedures could expose the musculoskeletal system to some acute injuries, such as knee and ankle sprains, joints' dislocations, muscle injuries and others. Moreover, some safety procedures are necessary to limit the risk of being hit by the car during pit stop manoeuvres. All these considerations justify the growing interest about the medical aspects of the Formula 1 World Championship. The motorsport in general is one of the sports in which safety has recently gained more relevance. Management and prevention of injuries are relevant topics in automobile sport. The safety of drivers and team members is mandatory and technical improvements are implemented continuously. Actually, FIA regulations include safety characteristics and safety checks, with the aim to limit driver and team member injuries in case of crashes. However, it is necessary to understand that injuries in the Formula 1 World Championship are not limited to car crashes and

to an acute involvement of the driver. Considering only this aspect of the problem could bias the real impact of injuries related to the Formula 1 World Championship. This concept is particularly relevant for health and medical personnel involved in the safety management during races organization. Therefore, health assistance in Formula 1 should be active on different settings and should be categorized in activities oriented to limit:

– Acute injuries in drivers and team members related to 'in competition' accidents.
– Chronic overuse musculoskeletal conditions in drivers.
– Chronic overuse musculoskeletal conditions in team members.

15.4 Epidemiology of Injuries in the Formula 1 World Championship

15.4.1 Acute Injuries in Drivers and Team Members Related to 'In Competition' Accidents

Each circuit involved in the Formula 1 World Championship is equipped with a medical centre to manage emergencies during race activities. An emerging interest of the FIA is the collection of data about accidents. For this reason, a Wold Accident Database (WADB) was instituted by FIA to collect data about serious accidents in Formula 1 and in other championships around the world. Data about characteristics of the accident are recorded (such as speed, acceleration, accident's description and medical consequences). The database includes data about Fatal Accidents (death occurs within 30 days of the accident), Serious Accidents (prognosis over 2 months), and Significant Accidents (when a vehicle involves a public area) [1]. This information should be relevant for event organizers, for engineers and for medical personnel, for preventing future accidents. Indeed, motorsport is strictly related to the accidents, and it is almost impossible to exclude accidents from motorsport completely. Nevertheless, it is possible to implement strategies to limit the consequence of race's accidents. Data from this database are analysed by FIA. Few published reports highlight injuries distribution among drivers during competition. In 2004, a report published in the British Journal of Sport Medicine reported an incidence rate of injury of 1.2 per 1000 competitors per race in a single-seat car competition. This rate was higher than incidence rate in saloon car competitions (0.9 per 1000 competitors per race). Data are not limited to the Formula 1 World Championship, but the characteristics of included competitions were similar. Bruises were the most common medical problems (58%), followed by neck sprain (34%). Abrasion, other sprain sites beyond neck region, concussion and death are reported less frequently (2% each). According to body region, the neck is the most involved region (34%) followed by lower limb (24%) and upper limb (14%) [2]. The entire body of the driver is hosted in the cockpit, while the neck and head are more exposed, being out of the cockpit. To prevent some head and neck trauma, a new specific device was introduced in 2018 as a mandatory system in each car: the HALO system. This structure serves to protect the drivers' head during accidents, and the analysis of previous accidents has shown its ability in increasing survival rate among drivers.

could be influenced by technical equipment in the vehicle and this could modify their incidence over the years. For example, a report about Formula 1 World Championship drivers in the 1998 season showed a high incidence of wrist problems (nervous symptoms as paraesthesia and osteoligamentousous damages) probably related to the large amount of vibrations, while incidence of these disorders in recent years seem to be reduced, due to some technical improvements. Another specific issue has to be taken into account when discussing chronic overuse effects on musculoskeletal system of drivers. Indeed, a professional driver starts his career in karting, passing through several championships to reach Formula 1. Drivers therefore start their career very young and, according to new FIA regulations, cannot participate in the Formula 1 World Championship before the age of 18 years old. During these years, drivers perform several championships spending several hours in less equipped vehicles and using simulators to learn circuits and strategies. It is notable that during these years, relevant forces act on a musculoskeletal system that is still growing.

Therefore, it is important to evaluate carefully musculoskeletal complaints in this population to avoid functional limitation during adolescence and adulthood.

15.4.2 Chronic Overuse Musculoskeletal Conditions in Drivers

Chronic exposure to vibration and G-forces lead to overuse injuries in the musculoskeletal system of drivers. Although direct data from Formula 1 World Championship drivers are not easily available, some cross-sectional observational study results showed complaints in the lumbar region, neck region and shoulder. Drivers' posture and comfort of seat seem to have a statistically significant association with musculoskeletal conditions in drivers [3]. Personalized seat in Formula 1, adaptation in cockpit and reduction of vibration could reduce symptoms in cervical spine and shoulders. Some musculoskeletal symptoms

15.4.3 Chronic Overuse Musculoskeletal Conditions in Team Members

Among team members, musculoskeletal complaints are relevant, representing the third cause of medical consultation after respiratory (i.e. upper respiratory tract inflammation) and gastrointestinal problems (i.e. nausea, vomiting and constipation). Traumatism in upper limbs are strictly connected to work activities (minor burns, skin abrasion, superficial cuts and others), but overuse musculoskeletal conditions are very frequent. The main musculoskeletal complaints are related to neck pain and low back pain. These conditions represent the main cause of referral for physiotherapy treatments. Load handling and prolonged postures are common risk factors for these musculoskeletal conditions. Radicular compressions should be noted among team members, but usually pain is related to contractures and spasms of paravertebral cervical and lumbar muscles. The other relevant musculoskeletal condition is represented by tendinopathies. Common anatomical sites involved are shoulders and elbows. Rotator cuff tendinopathy and epicondylitis are common among mechanics. Sometimes, they are directly related to specific activities such as the prolonged used of some equipment such as screwdrivers, hex keys and others or wheel guns used during pit stops, forcing upper limbs to control movements against a high-pressure demand.

15.5 Diagnostic Imaging in Formula 1

Current diagnostic imaging technology provides highly accurate information on the most common musculoskeletal conditions affecting Formula 1 drivers through a variety of approaches.

15.5.1 Equipment and Methods

Diagnostic imaging can rely on a wide range of methods. Conventional radiography, computed tomography, ultrasound elastography (USE) and static and dynamic magnetic resonance imaging (MRI) with the patient lying down or standing up are the most commonly used techniques.

USE and, especially, dynamic upright MRI (Fig. 15.1) supply highly accurate images that afford optimal assessment of the body's biomechanics. The information processed by USE software is translated into a colour scale depicting the degree of elasticity of the different tissues (e.g. muscle, tendon, ligament), which ranges from soft (elastic tissue) to hard (stiffer tissue), using a qualitative (strain) and a quantitative (share wave) method. Upright MRI and dynamic functional MRI provide realistic images under stress loading. The main pathological conditions involving the cervical spine of Formula 1 drivers,

with the obvious exception of accident-related trauma, are reviewed below.

15.5.2 Cervical Spine Injuries

The most common conditions affecting Formula 1 drivers are induced by their rigid, forced posture in the cockpit and by the strong lateral G-forces to which they are exposed, which involve constant contraction of muscles and capsuloligamentous components. Lateral and flexion-extension scanning using dynamic upright MRI is the most suitable approach to investigate the state of muscles, tendons and capsuloligamentous structures. At our diagnostic centre, with the assistance of Fabrizio Borra, pilots undergo dynamic MRI in flexion-extension in the sagittal plane with and without a HANS device, to measure the excursion of their cervical spine (Fig. 15.2). The investigation is completed by dynamic USE, which supplies an accurate evaluation of the contraction of each muscle component, especially the sternocleidomastoid and paravertebral muscles (Fig. 15.3). Owing to the typically high loads to which drivers are exposed, we recommend serial monitoring of the larger vertebral hemangiomas.

Examination of the greater occipital nerve is important because this nerve is often affected by acute and chronic conditions involving the cervical spine. A thorough examination includes dynamic ultrasound, colour and power Doppler sonography and USE and is completed by a dynamic MRI scan.

The chronic strain sustained by the cervical spine often induces formation of large protrusions, which besides functional imaging must be investigated by dynamic MRI in flexion-extension in the sagittal plane, to determine the degree of stenosis of the spinal canal (Fig. 15.4).

In patients with suspected low-lying cerebellar tonsils or frank Chiari I malformation, especially those with syringomyelia, we recommend dynamic and upright MRI assessment also with the Valsalva manoeuvre.

Fig. 15.1 (**a** and **b**)
Dynamic MRI of the
lumbar spine in supine
(0°) and weight-bearing
(80°) position.

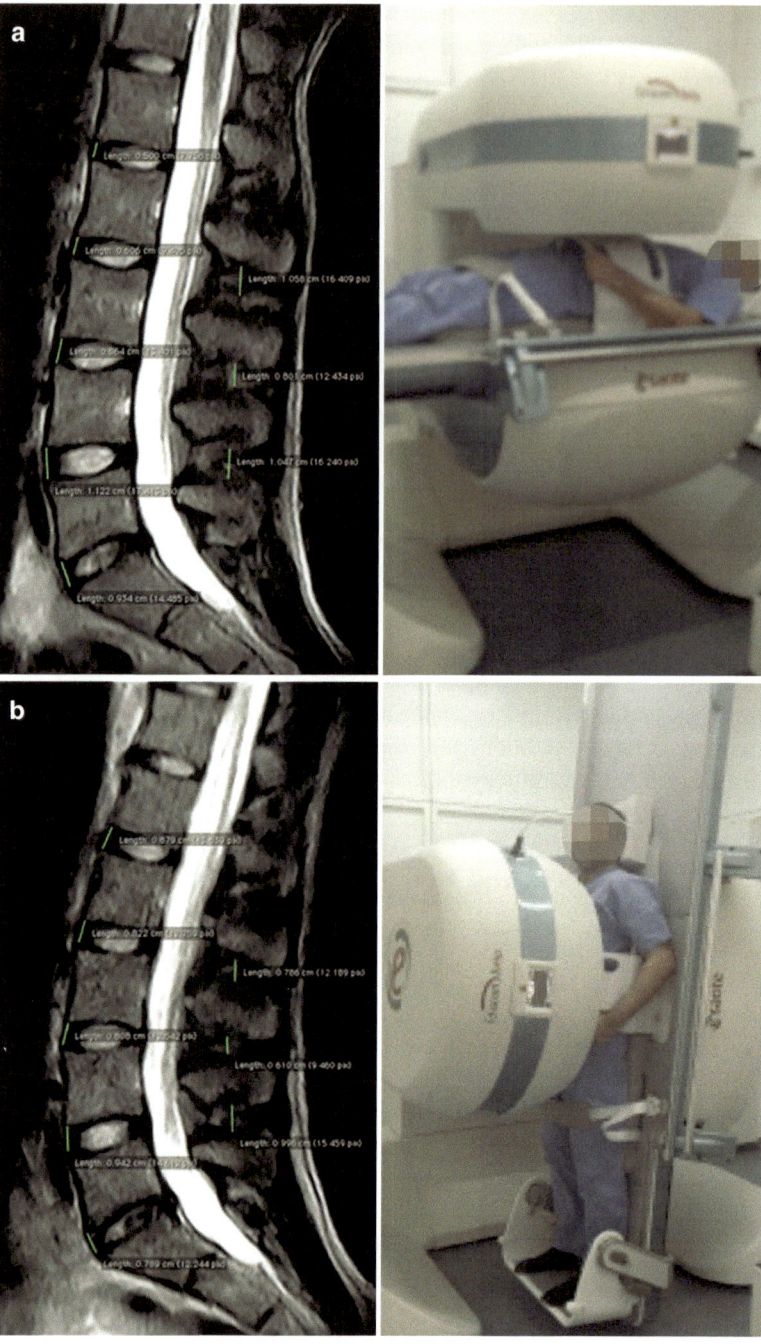

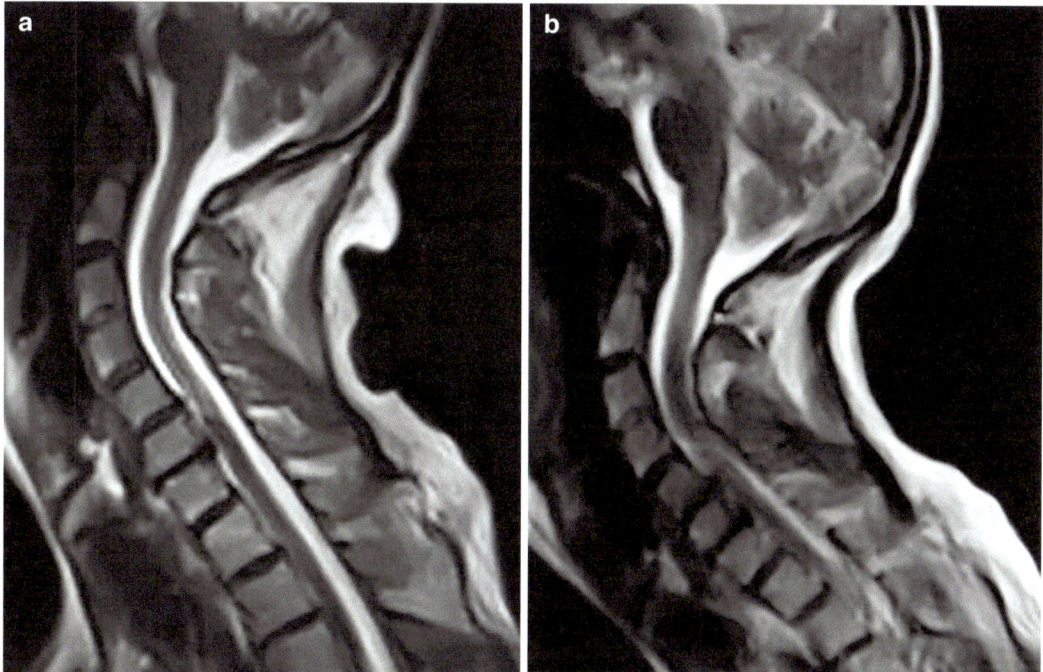

Fig. 15.2 Frames of dynamic MRI at the cervical level, performed without (**a**) and with (**b**) Hans' collar

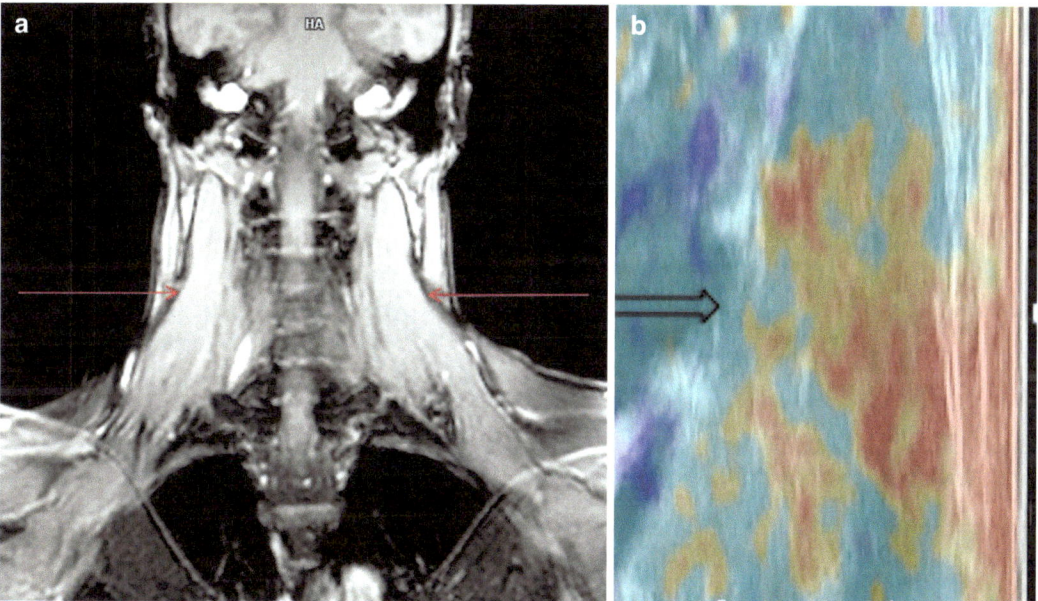

Fig. 15.3 Dynamic study of the sternocleidomastoid muscle performed with dynamic MRI (**a**) and USE (**b**), where marked contracture is highlighted

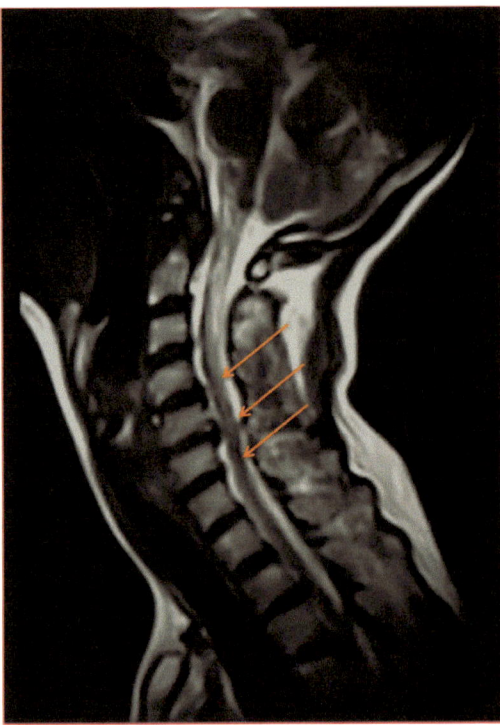

Fig. 15.4 Dynamic MRI in maximum anterior flexion highlights the multiple herniated discs

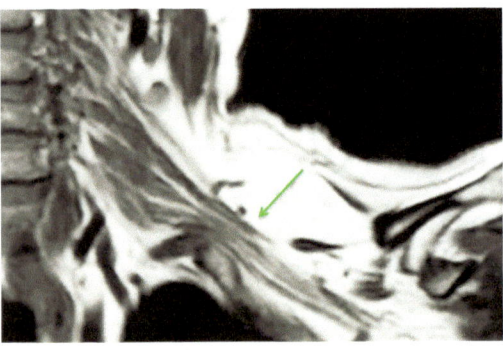

Fig. 15.5 Dynamic and orthostatic MRI demonstrates evident compression of the brachial plexus cords that cannot otherwise be demonstrated with investigation in supine position

The differential diagnosis of cervical spine pain includes temporomandibular joint conditions and post-traumatic oropharyngeal dysphagia.

The continuous vibration characteristic of Formula 1 cars, due to the rigid chassis, has the potential to affect the vascular and nerve structures of the brachial plexus, for instance, induc-

ing an enlargement of the seventh cervical transverse process at the level of the thoracic outlet, which may go undetected (Fig. 15.5).

Dynamic MRI performed with the patient lying down, standing and in the inverted posture enables accurate examination of the diaphragm, especially in patients who have sustained contusion traumas, which often involve the phrenic nerve (Fig. 15.6).

The small cockpit can also be responsible for hematomas due to para- and pericostal contusion, which is clearly depicted by MRI, especially on dynamic and upright scans.

Evaluation of the correct posture of the lumbar spine is also essential, because if the loading axis is not held very straight (90°), the load on L3, which is the fulcrum of this tract, increases exponentially. A typical consequence of incorrect lumbar posture is anterolisthesis, which is responsible for severe pain and instability, especially in the forced sitting posture of Formula 1 drivers (Fig. 15.7).

These athletes may also develop a grossly hypertrophic quadratus femoris muscle, which often induces severe sciatic pain; during muscle contraction this condition may mimic disc herniation.

Pain in the ischiocrural region is optimally investigated by dynamic MRI of the sacroiliac joint, which is frequently unstable and is responsible for severe pain, with the patient standing on one or both feet.

Finally, symptoms involving joints such as the shoulder, elbow, wrist and knee, where continuous friction and impacts against the small cockpit can result in reactive bursitis or tenosynovitis, can be evaluated by dynamic ultrasound.

15.6 Rehabilitation and Return to Play

The technical specialization among team members is very high and selective. Therefore, each injury could determine the exclusion of a team member with peculiar technical skills within the organizational process of activities about the vehicle. Therefore, the substitution of team

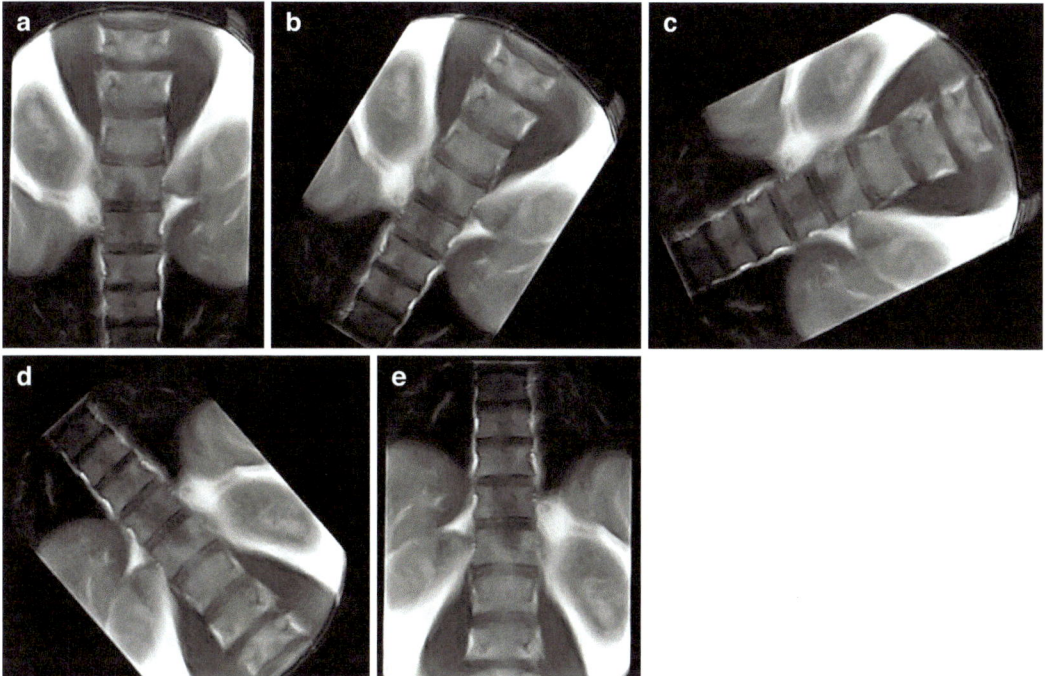

Fig. 15.6 Dynamic study of the diaphragm muscle performed overturning at 60° (**a, b, c, d, e**), fundamental in the evaluation of chest trauma

members is not easy. From this point of view, return to play becomes a crucial point in the rehabilitation phase of injuries in the Formula 1 World Championship. Owing to the close events in the calendar, it is almost impossible to plan an 'in home' rehabilitation process for injuries. For this reason, some teams include a medical doctor and a physiotherapist among team members and a dedicated temporary medical room in the box or in the hospitality facilities. In this way, each complaint should be assessed by medical doctor acutely and managed according to local health regulations. If the medical condition is defined as stabilized and not harmful, pharmacological treatment should be appropriately delivered. It is necessary to take into consideration that some drugs commonly used in musculoskeletal conditions are considered as doping agents in sports (i.e. oral administration or intramuscular injections of steroids). Therefore, WADA (World Anti-Doping Agency) list consultation is mandatory before starting any pharmacological treatment in drivers [4]. In more complex situations, the patient is referred to race medical centre. If a musculoskeletal

problem is diagnosed and a physiotherapy approach is considered appropriate, a series of treatments are planned during the week of the race. This approach is carried out worldwide by doctors and physiotherapists that follow the team during the events.

15.6.1 Neck Pain and Low Back Pain in Drivers

Acute onset of neck and low back pain in drivers during the race or free proofs should be assessed carefully. Sometimes symptoms could begin without a crash or accident. Some drivers experience an acute neck or low back pain while driving, especially during some high-degree high-velocity turns. In this case, it is essential to exclude some radicular or spinal involvement. Localization of pain is carefully detected, putting more attention on painful symptoms referred on median line or exacerbated by vertebral spinous process compression. Sensory symptoms are assessed in upper and lower limbs, to exclude an acute onset of paresthesia, dysesthesia or hypoes-

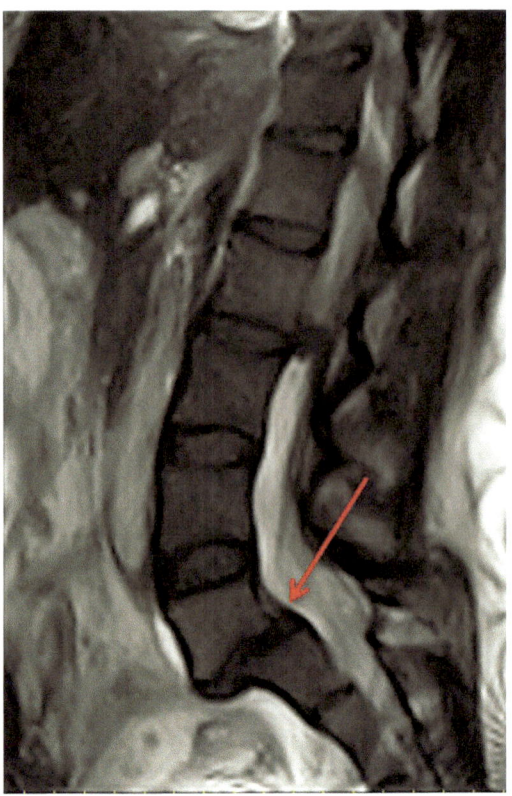

Fig. 15.7 Orthostatic study of a L5-S1 anterolisthesis picture which is markedly accentuated in dynamics, especially in comparison to MR in supine position

thesia/anesthesia. Passive range of motion in several planes of the space is assessed gently. Active movements against gravity and manual resistance are performed to investigate segmental strength. If sensory symptoms, marked passive movement limitation or segmental weakness are detected, the driver is referred to the medical centre for more investigations. If a muscular origin of the pain is detected, with active trigger points within paravertebral muscles, a physiotherapy approach is carried out to reduce muscle spasms and contractions. Usually, hot packs, massage, manual mobilization and active exercises are performed to reduce pain and increase range of motion.

15.6.2 Shoulder in Drivers

In Formula 1 World Championship's drivers, the shoulder joint is required to manage a high func-tional demand. Prolonged posture in the cockpit, with limited rotational movements to control the vehicle, is required during the race. Nevertheless, thoraco-appendicular muscles and scapular muscles are required to sustain prolonged isometric contractions to control movement accurately. This functional demand involves prolonged tension applied to tendons of the rotator cuff. Among them, the supraspinatus tendon is commonly involved in drivers, with partial tears. Sometimes, fluid is collected within an inflamed subacromion-subdeltoid bursa configuring a painful bursitis able to limit shoulder movements. This painful condition limits the ability to drive. Passive movements are usually limited, especially in flexion, abduction and external rotation. Impingement tests are commonly performed (i.e. Jobe's test, Yocum's test, Neer's test). Segmental strength, especially in external rotation is assessed to evaluate tendons' function. Shoulder stability should be evaluated in several directions. A physiotherapy approach commonly includes: active and passive exercises to reduce tendon's impingement; exercise to recover the range of motion; kinesiotaping application. Some tendinopathies are treated with physical therapy as extracorporeal shock-waves therapy, available in some medical rooms worldwide during the races. Elastic resistance exercise are performed easily in the medical room, under doctor and physiotherapist supervision.

15.6.3 Tendinopathy in Team Members

Tendinopathy is a common problem among team members involved in the assembly of the vehicles. Indeed, a large number of procedures require manual intervention to configure the different sections of the vehicle correctly. Some work areas are particularly restricted and require maintaining forced postures. Holding these postures, a high level of strength is produced by forearm and hand muscles. Moreover, these movements are repeated hundreds of times during consecutive days. As a result, an overuse involvement of tendons occurs. The most common anatomical site involved is the common extensor tendon in the elbow, with bone attachment localized to humeral lateral epicondyle.

Diagnosis is easily performed through some clinical tests such as Cozen test and Chair test. Segmental strength of forearm and hand muscles should always be addressed to exclude the involvement of peripheral nervous structures (i.e. posterior interosseous nerve). Ice packs are applied in the painful region, with a gentle massage. Some manual therapy techniques are performed in the painful region, i.e. deep friction massage. Although contrasting results exist about the use of orthosis, it is commonly encouraged considering the prolonged exposure of these tendons to sustained and repetitive stress. Kinesiotaping is commonly performed, such as extracorporeal shock-waves therapy. Eccentric exercises are planned, illustrated to the patient and performed with doctor and physiotherapist supervision.

15.6.4 Joints Disorders in Team Members

Several activities around the car are performed while working under it or to its side. For team members this implies to adopt a forced and prolonged posture on the knees. Moreover, during some high-demand activities such as pit-stops, members acting on the tyres are on the knees or have to manage tyres in an unstable position pushing the tyre forward towards the car. These procedures determine a high functional demand on some joint's structures. Commonly knee joints are involved. Inflammatory processes of this joint manifest with knee effusion and an increase of skin temperature over the knee.

Reduction in passive and active flexion is common and particularly limiting for the patient, with limitation in squat movement. Sometimes, prolonged periods of rest are difficult to plan during the week of the race. For these reasons, ice-packs are adopted several times during a day, for 20–30 min. Manual massage is carried out to reduce effusion and to increase range of movement. Some exercises are performed to preserve and limit muscle hypotrophy, especially in the muscles of the anterior compartment of the thigh.

15.7 Prevention Strategies

To plan prevention strategies limiting injuries in the Formula 1 World Championship is the most reasonable approach. Some prevention strategies are useful on track for driver's safety. Some other devices are integrated in the vehicles to detect conditions that could potentially harm the driver, such as an excessive increase in G–force. According to FIA regulations, some devices are mandatory for drivers. Helmets have to respond to some specific characteristics of resistance to crash and should have limited opening to admit vision comfortably. A HANS device (Hand and Neck Support) is adopted by all drivers. This device holds the helmet to a specific support over the shoulders of drivers. In the case of deceleration, this device prevents the excessive flexion of the cervical spine. Indeed, through HANS, some forces are directed to the dorsal spine and the entire trunk is forced to flex, avoiding extreme cervical spine flexion that could damage the cervical spine. Belts prevent excessive body movements within the cockpit. Specific pilot suits are designed to be light and fireproof. Within the box, organizational strategies among team members are useful to limit risks related to work activity. During assembly of the box, a lot of material is organized and prepared for the race. These activities include the use of working vehicles or mobilization of voluminous cases. The assembly and disassembly of the box, indeed, represses the most dangerous phases in a single race for team members' safety. During these activities, coordination of the operations is essential. Each team member is designated to perform a specific task. During the races over the year, standardization procedures are implemented to reduce the time for these operations and to make these processes more efficient.

Beyond these organizational safety aspects, some medical procedures are adopted during the whole year in some teams ('In Season' prevention strategies) and other activities are designed to prevent musculoskeletal disorders during the race ('In Race' prevention strategies).

15.7.1 'In Season' Prevention Strategies

Some teams organize a medical check-up activity for their members. This could include a complete cardiovascular assessment (history, physical examination, rest ECG, spirometry, exercise stress tests and cardiac ultrasound). Anthropometric data are used to calculate indexes such as body mass index. Bioimpedentiometry was performed to measure fat mass, muscle mass, body water and composition within the body. Abdominal ultrasound and colour-Doppler ultrasound of upper and lower limbs is performed. Eye, otolaryngology, nutritional and dermatological evaluations are carried out. Postural assessment and musculoskeletal evaluation were performed by a physiatrist. Several fitness tests are conducted to assess strength in upper limbs (dynamometer) and lower limbs (accelerometer). Reaction times are relevant in this motor sport and are assessed trough several specific devices. Flexibility is assessed by sit-and-reach test [5]. Throughout the season, team members are invited to repeat fitness tests and to participate in a physical educational programme to improve the most deficient functions.

15.7.2 'In Race' Prevention Strategies

Some strategies have been adopted to limit injuries during the races. Changing several time zones in a short period could lead to sleep disturbances. This could cause several dysfunctions in different systems and mechanisms within the body with cognitive, hormonal, gastrointestinal and other effects able to interfere with work activities. Moreover, sometimes these disturbances are treated with drugs affecting attention and concentration. Therefore, specific educational programmes have been promoted to limit jet lag effects such as avoid alcohol consumption during the flight, limit the use of stimulants such as caffeine, plan sleeping hours according to flight destination and others.

A sufficient hydration is recommended. Nutritional advertisements are provided to team members, avoiding food with high-fat concentration. Moreover, the menu during the races is planned according to medical staff to limit the intake of food able to negatively interfere with performance. Physical activity is promoted at the end of the working time. Under the supervision of the physiotherapist, voluntary groups of runners, among team members, are organized to complete a lap of the track or to run across trails nearby, according to the location of the race. Some teams organize dedicated sections of physical activity using the fitness centres of the hotels where the team members stay. Importantly, an increasing number of teams provide a specific warm up programme before pit-stop practice and before the race. Indeed, each team tests pit-stop procedures several times to standardize them and to try to perform them as fast as possible. However, this activity requires a high musculoskeletal involvement. For this reason, a restricted set of exercises are performed before the session of pit-stop, including aerobic exercises, dynamic stretching, elastic resistance exercises, reaction activation exercises and specific task-oriented exercises according to the procedure performed in the pit-stop from each specific team member.

References

1. FIA – World Accident. Database. 2020; https://www.fia.com/wadb-world-accident-database. Accessed 12 January 2020
2. Minoyama O, Tsuchida H. Injuries in professional motor car racing drivers at a racing circuit between 1996 and 2000. Br J Sports Med. 2004;38:613–6.
3. Koutras C, Buecking B, Jaeger M, Ruchholtz S, Heep H. Musculoskeletal Injuries in Auto Racing: A Retrospective Study of 137 Drivers. Phys Sportsmed. 2014;42:80–6.
4. WADA (World Anti-Doping Agency) prohibited list (2020). https://www.wada-ama.org/en/resources/science-medicine/prohibited-list-documents. Accessed 12 January 2020.
5. Biffi A, Fernando F, Adami PE, Messina M, Sirico F, Di Paolo F, et al. Ferrari Corporate Wellness Program: Results of a Pilot Analysis and the "Drag" Impact in the Workplace. High Blood Press Cardiovasc Prev. 2018 Sep;25(3):261–6.

Motocross

16

Alberto Gobbi and Giacomo Valsecchi

16.1 Characteristics of Motocross

Motocross is a high speed competition, which is conducted based on the engine class of the motorcycle. All the riders are lined up at the start and drive along an uneven 2 km circuit as fast as possible for a fixed time of 30–40 min. The track is usually made of natural terrain with dirt, mud, sharp turns, and steep hills that allow the driver to perform jumps that can reach 20 m in length and 5 m in height [1]. The competition consists of two or three "matches" with a short break between them.

Enduro races take place over country roads, mule tracks, and public streets under ordinary traffic rules. These routes are unknown to the riders and therefore it is easy for them to encounter unexpected obstacles and unmarked roads. The distance between several checkpoints must be covered within a fixed time (i.e., within a fixed average speed), stressing endurance rather than speed. Along the track there are sometimes trials from 4 to 10 km long that must be covered as fast as possible. The competition usually lasts 6–8 h and the final result is calculated as the sum of the times of the trials and the penalties owing to the differences between the fixed required time and the real time spent covering the track.

Rally is a staged race under ordinary traffic rules that keeps the rider busy for several days (up to 20 days) on a route that is thousands of kilometers long (the Paris–Dakar race reached the length of 14,000 km). In rally the riders must follow the route with the help of a road book given at the start of the competition. Desert areas and wild, uninhabited places are often crossed. In this context, unexpected troubles from the motorcycle or other causes could have tragic consequences.

16.2 Physiological and Biomechanical Demands of Motocross Riders

As far as motor sports are concerned, research has always been focused on improving the technical aspects of a bike such as engine efficiency, suspension, etc., while the rider is generally considered to be important only for technical or tactical tasks. Often, the physiological characteristics of the rider are generally over looked as a contributing factor in the overall performance of the rider. However, during a competitive off-road motorsport racing, the understanding about physiological demands of the rider plays an important role during training and injury prevention.

A. Gobbi (✉) · G. Valsecchi
Orthopaedic Arthroscopic Surgery International Bioresearch Foundation NPO, Milan, Italy
e-mail: gobbi@cartilagedoctor.it

© The Author(s), under exclusive license to Springer-Verlag GmbH, DE, part of Springer Nature 2022
G. L. Canata, H. Jones (eds.), *Epidemiology of Injuries in Sports*,
https://doi.org/10.1007/978-3-662-64532-1_16

In our previous published study [2], the physiological characteristics of top level riders participating in three different types of off-road motorcycling (motocross, enduro, and desert rally) were analyzed to facilitate the development of specific training programs. The results showed that motocross riders have more muscle mass, higher strength, and greater aerobic power and physical attributes, which enhance their ability to effectively maximize the mechanical and technical capabilities of modern motorcycles. Based on the results, we found that these motorcycling sports require active involvement of the entire musculoskeletal system with aerobic metabolism maintained at a level slightly above the anaerobic threshold. Hence, determination of the difference in the physical morphology of riders becomes more important in designing a well-structured specific training program, improving the rider's ability to withstand the rigorous competition.

In our study [2], the motocross and enduro riders were found to be at the highest limit for normal values for weight, while rally riders tended to be overweight. The latter also have, on average, a higher percentage of adipose tissue in comparison to the top level athletes practicing other sports, such as distance running, cycling, cross-country skiing, volleyball, and basketball. In motor sports, being overweight is a negative factor due to increase in the load for the bike as well as extra mass that must be accelerated and decelerated during braking. Hence, the heavier athletes required more muscular force for the optimal control of their motorcycle. In addition, we found that the rally rider may have a little higher percentage of adipose tissue (between 13 and 16%), which might be considered as energy reserve and consequently a positive factor for performance.

As far as motocross is concerned, the intense competition and the frequent changes of direction and speed owing to the nature of the circuit require constant involvement of all the muscle groups in the body. Therefore, they involve both aerobic and lactic acid metabolisms, which correlates with our finding of, the maximum aerobic power in the motocross riders compared to sedentary people ($p < 0.01$) and to the rally and enduro riders ($p < 0.001$). Moreover, the motocross riders have more involvement of the upper extremities, which increases the aerobic power in comparison to the enduro and rally riders.

The handgrip strength was similar in the three groups of athletes. It is well known that in sedentary subjects there is a significant difference in handgrip strength between the dominant and non-dominant limb. Maughan et al. reported that in untrained subjects, these differences presumably reflect the greater use of the dominant arm in normal daily activities [4]. However, in motocross, the left arm, which was the non-dominant arm in all the subjects, was significantly stronger than the right arm (+6%, $p < 0.05$). These differences may be the result of constant use of the clutch lever with the left hand, which is more frequently used in motocross compared to enduro and rally riders.

In motocross riders, heart rate is generally higher than 80% of the maximum theoretical heart rate, and it is maintained at quite high levels throughout the duration of the race. On the other hand, in enduro and rally riders, the heart rate was generally lower (20–50% of maximum heart rate) and tends to increase during the most difficult parts of the track, but only for a few minutes.

Blood lactate concentrations at the end of the races show a different involvement of the anaerobic metabolism. In motocross, blood lactate concentrations resulted in significantly higher values than in enduro and rally ($p < 0.01$). According to Relly and Secher, it is possible to classify motocross among the sports with mixed aerobic–anaerobic demands, while enduro and rally are mainly aerobic. The lactate accumulation is related to the fatigue that typically occurs with intensive exercise leading to a feeling of "tiredness" or fatigue in their limbs. This fatigue, especially in motocross, is mainly due to the static involvement of several muscle groups and produces a decrease in muscular force that is necessary to oppose the negative and the positive accelerations of the engine during the race. Therefore, it is impossible to obtain the best performance of the motorcycle when the maximum force is required. This state of fatigue is one of the human factors that may limit the performance in motor sports and must be considered during training.

16.2.1 Incidence of Motocross Injuries

In our previous study [1], we analyzed a group of 15,870 athletes participating in European off-road competitions (11,902 outdoor and 3968 indoor) at different levels for a 12 year period. There were 1500 (905 outdoor and 595 indoor) accidents involving rider injuries; the data was used to classify and locate the injuries, as well as the modality of the accidents, protective gear used, and the recovery.

The overall incidence of accidents was 94.5% per year for motocross races, which is significantly lower than the 115% for road races; furthermore, the incidence of accidents in the stadium cross competitions was significantly higher at 150% per year than outdoor motocross, which was only around 76%.

Among the total of 1870 injuries, there were 450 fractures (50.9% in the upper, 38% in the lower extremity) (Table 16.1), and the rest were on the spine, chest, and skull. The 26 spine fractures (5.8%) produced permanent neurologic sequelae in eight patients.

Ligamentous lesions accounted for 344 cases with 206 (59.9%) occurring in the lower extremities, especially on the knee (42.4%). Head trauma was noted in 86 cases (5.7% of accidents) producing coma in 3%, and loss of consciousness in 14%. It was concluded that motocross is a high-risk sport and despite the reduction of some injuries by better protective gear (helmet, chest protector, neck, knee, and wrist braces) the occurrence of these lesions remains high. Moreover, when compared with soccer, the overall injury rate is 3.6 times higher in motocross [5].

16.2.2 Basic Rules of Injury Prevention

In a study conducted by Tomida et al. [5], the injury rate in motocross sport is 22.4 per 1000 h, which is 3.6 times higher than that of soccer. Primary prevention includes measures that can be taken prior to the occurrence of the injury such as appropriate training, protective gear, maintenance of the vehicle, and environmental factors. Secondary prevention aims to minimize the consequences after the injury (first aid, transfer to a specialized center, follow-up care).

16.2.2.1 Rider Protection

Protective devices worn by a motocross rider during a race are important in order to avoid injuries. Clothing must meet three main requirements:

1. Protect the vital parts on hitting the ground;
2. Protect the face from stones and dirt thrown up by riders in front;
3. Fabrics should allow good transpiration with minimum weight and encumbrance.

Usage of protective equipment such as helmet, goggles, chestguard, kidney belt, fire retardant trousers, boots, gauntlets, vest with elbow pads,

Table 16.1 Motocross injuries according to type and location of lesion

Type of lesion	Location of lesion							
	Upper extremity	Lower extremity	Face	Skull	Cranium (including concussions)	Chest	Spine	Total
Fractures (450)	229 (50.9%)	171 (38.0%)	0	10 (2.2%)	–	14 (3.1%)	26 (5.8%)	450 (24.1%)
Sprains and dislocations (344)	138 (40.1%)	206 (59.9%)	–	–	–	–	–	344 (18.4%)
Contusion and abrasions (1076)	300 (27.9%)	290 (26.9%)	172 (16%)	–	86 (8%)	228 (21.2%)	0	1076 (57.5%)
Total	667	667	172	10	86	242	26	1870

knee braces, neck braces, and elbow pads can help a rider to evade a disabling or life threatening injury.

16.3 Conclusion

Motocross is a high risk sport and is today's most widely practiced motorcycle sport, both in Europe and the USA. Some injuries such as maxillofacial and skull injuries, knee and ankle sprain, and wrist fractures have been reduced by better protective gear and hopefully neck sprains and fractures will be on the downswing with newer braces and helmets. Unlike soccer where most of the injury prevention happens off-field, injury prevention in motocross can be sought through better equipment, riding techniques, physical training, and limited access to minors.

We believe that increasing involvement of the physician with competitive riders and the evolution of training methods will lead to making this sport much safer for the motorcyclists.

References

1. Gobbi A, Tuy B, Panuncialman I. The incidence of motocross injuries: a 12-year investigation. Knee Surg Sports Traumatol Arthrosc. 2004;12:574–80.
2. Gobbi A, Francisco R, Tuy B, et al. Physiological characteristics of top level off-road motorcyclists. Br J Sports Med. 2005;39:927–93.
3. Maughan RJ, Abel RW, Watson JS, Weir J. Forearm composition and muscle function in trained and untrained limbs. Clin Physiol. 1986;6:389–96.
4. Gobbi A. The incidence of motocross injuries. J Sports Traumatol Rel Res. 1992;14:241–8.
5. Tomida Y, Hirata H, Fukuda A, et al. Injuries in elite motorcycle racing in Japan. Br J Sports Med. 2005;39:508–11.

Rugby

17

Michael R. Carmont,
Pierfilippo Bottiglia Amici Grossi, Luca Pulici,
Francois Kelberine, and Catherine Lester

17.1 Characteristics of the Sport

Rugby is a popular contact collision sport played worldwide. In 2014, there were more than 6 million people playing, of whom 2.36 million were registered players. In 1845, the first football laws were written by Rugby School pupils, when allegedly William Webb Ellis picked up a football and ran with it. The sport of rugby became distinct from football when Blackheath Club left the Football Association in 1863. The sport was always considered amateur; however players in some pro-

M. R. Carmont (✉)
Department of Trauma and Orthopaedic Surgery, Princess Royal Hospital, Shrewsbury and Telford Hospital NHS Trust, Shropshire, UK

P. B. A. Grossi
Clinica Ortopedica, ASST Centro Specialistico Ortopedico Traumatologico Gaetano Pini-CTO, Milan, Italy

L. Pulici
Knee Surgery and Sport Traumatology Unit, Humanitas Research Hospital, Milan, Italy

F. Kelberine
Pôle Aixois de Chirurgie Articulaire et Sportive, Aix en Provence, France

C. Lester
Pure Sports Medicine, Moving Medicine, Northampton Saints, Northampton, UK

fessions suffered financial hardship by having to take unpaid time off from work to play. Discussions regarding payment in lieu for these players occurred at the George Hotel in Huddersfield, England, on the 29th August 1895 to the formation of the Northern Rugby Football Union. Over the next 15 years many clubs left the Rugby Football Union to form what became known as the Rugby Football League. The first world cup in rugby was the Rugby League World Cup held in 1954. Since then the competition has been held every 2–8 years. In the Union code the Rugby World Cup was first held in 1987 and consists of a tournament of 20 nations. A seven-a-side union game is contested at the Commonwealth Games and was first contested in the 1900 Olympic Games in Paris.

Both codes have similar rules in that the oval shaped ball must be touched on the ground on or over the try line to score a try. A subsequent place kick, level with the place at which the try was scored, allows a conversion for further points if the ball goes over the horizontal crossbar of the posts. The ball may be carried forward or kicked forward but may only be passed backward. Only the ball carrier may be tackled, or stopped by wrapping the tackler's arms around the body or legs of the ball carrier. There is no limit to the amount of force that may be applied but a tackled player may not be lifted up and forced into the ground (spear tackle).

Once forward progression has been stopped, in Union the ball must be released backwards to maintain possession. The opposing team may be able to reach over the tackled player to retrieve a loose ball but their feet must not leave the ground, without kneeling. In League six tackles are permitted before possession of the ball is exchanged. Both codes have scrums to permit restart after minor infringements. In a scrum the forwards are bound together and link with the opposition. In League, scrums remove forwards from open play giving more room for the unoccupied field of play. In Union the scrum is contested and both packs push against each other aiming to move forwards, after the ball has been put in between them. In open play the ball may be kicked over the crossbar of the posts to score a drop goal. If a penalty is awarded further points can be scored by the succession of the ball from a place kick over the crossbar. A game or match lasts 80 min, split into halves of 40 min separated by 15 min.

17.2 Physiological and Biomechanical Demands on Athletes

Athletes in all sports now are stronger, faster and bigger than they were 15 years ago. When you add all this strength, power and speed together, you have the potential for more serious injuries.

The forces applied to opposing players are considerable akin to a car crash or collision between charging musk oxen; however engagement techniques and playing position have a considerable role in the impact during simulated scrummaging. Additionally specific coaching may be required for non-dominant side tackling. Studies have shown that there is considerable fluctuation in the running demands of players from any position during the game. This is except for full backs who demonstrated greater running intensity. The intensity of running performed is usually short-distance sprint performance generating high levels of horizontal force and power.

17.3 Epidemiology of Injuries

Rugby is a collective contact collision sport so it increases dramatically forces of injury. As a consequence injuries occur at all levels of the sport from international to youth community participants. The risk factors for injury in ball carriers are at their highest during high tackles, with high speed, increased impact force and head-to-head contact. Tacklers have a greater risk of head injuries with head-to-head contact resulting in the greatest number of head injuries. Based on position backs have greater risk of head injury when tackling compared to forwards.

Overall injuries occur during matches at the highest rate with 91 injuries/1000 player hours, giving on average 18 days' time lost. Thigh injuries are more common in forwards, and ACL and hamstring injuries in backs. The majority occur during contact with only 18% injuries as a result of foul play. On average a club will have 18% of players unavailable as a consequence of match injuries.

Injuries occur much less frequently during training, 2 per 1000 player hours, but tend to be more severe with greater time away from sport >24 days lost. Forwards sustain mainly lumbar disc/nerve root and shoulder dislocation or instability. The back players sustain ACL injuries (29% of days missed), MCL injuries (25% days missed) or hamstring injuries (0.27/1000 player hours during training compared with 5.6/1000 h during match play, 17 days' time lost). Each club will suffer from 10 knee injuries per season.

In a prospective five-season study of South African Super Rugby Tournament the rate of match injury was higher than most elite or international series with 93.2 match injuries per 1000 player hours. 39.8% of players in Super Rugby were injured at some point in 2016. Contact (79%) and tackle (54%) were the most common mechanisms of injury.

Risk of injury in international rugby is significantly lower for women than men, with 35.5/1000 player hours; tackle is the cause of most injuries similarly to the male game. A systematic review of 10 studies reporting injuries in women's rugby reported that injuries in the 15 s game peaked at 19.6 per 1000 match hours; however, the 7 s game had a much higher rate of 62.5 per 1000 match hours. In Collegiate women's rugby the rate was approximately half that in the Women's Rugby World Cup of 5.5 compared to 11.8 per 1000 h of match play. The incidence of injury in female 15 s and 7 s rugby is comparable to that in male youth 15 s rugby [1].

Epidemiological studies of an international U-20 tournament have revealed an incidence of 49.7/1000 player match hours with an average severity of 32.2 days' absence per injury. This indicated a high rate of injury but was approximately half that of senior level [2].

17.3.1 Anatomical Injury Patterns

Shoulder injuries occur with 8.9/1000 player hours during matches and much less during training 0.1/1000 player hours. The most common injury is acromio-clavicular joint injury of 32%, whereas the most severe is a glenohumeral joint dislocation resulting in 81 days' absence. The outside backs are most likely to sustain an injury occurring in 2.4/100 player tackles. Training resulted in the most severe injuries with an absence of 61 days with defensive training sessions having the highest risk injury of 0.45/1000 player hours. Shoulder injuries resulted in a mean 241 player days lost per season.

Regarding the cervical spine, 42% of injuries occur in the scrum, tackle 34%, rucks and mauls 20% and other phases of the game 4%. The incidence of cervical spine injuries is 1–2/100,000 per year. For spinal injuries overall, match play consists of 10.9/1000 player hours causing predominantly the cervical nerve root and in training 0.37/1000 player hours predominantly affecting the lumbar discs. The scrum accounts for 6–8% of all injuries but 41% of front-row spinal injuries at 10/1000 player hours at elite level compared to 2/1000 player hours at youth level.

Head injury is relatively common with 6.6 injuries/1000 player hours per match, and con-

cussion occurs at a rate of 4.1 concussions/1000 h making it the third most common injury for all match play. Concussion reflects a functional rather than structural injury and standard neuro-imaging is typically normal. Most concussions are sustained from tackling head on 28%, and next due to collisions, 20%. On average, a professional rugby union player is more likely than not to sustain a concussion after 25 matches and players have a 60% greater risk of time loss due to injury after concussion. In rugby union in Ireland the rate of concussion during match play was 18.4 per 1000 player match hours providing a burden of 5 days of absence from the team for each concussion [3]. Players who sustained a single concussion are six times more likely to sustain another concussion in their entire career and three times in the same season [4, 5]. Rugby players with a history of two or more concussions have reduced neuropsychological testing; the domain that is affected most is visuomotor processing speed [6].

The brain health of players following retirement from the game has been studied using a systematic review. Six studies of moderate quality reported a subjective increase in subjective cognitive complaints with persistent post-concussion symptoms associated with a higher number of self-reported concussions and decreased fine motor control [7]. Former rugby players reported distress (11%), anxiety and depression (28%), sleep disturbance (12%) and adverse alcohol use (22%). For 46% of players specific support measures were not available [8].

Catastrophic or severe injuries are rare with 1.8–7.9 per 100,000 players [9].

In foot and ankle injuries, an injury to the lateral ligament complex is the most common; however Achilles tendon ruptures account for more than half of absence due to injury. The incidence is highest in second row forwards. Stress fractures in the foot account for 8% of fractures and navicular stress fractures account for the longest absence of 188 days.

Rugby union when played in the seven-a-side format has a higher still incidence of injury with injuries occurring at 133/1000 h of play, with a severity of 22.22 days. 81.5% of these occurred during contact with most affecting the lower limb (66.7%) [10]. In the World Sevens series 2008–2009 an injury incidence of 106.1/1000 player hours was reported suggesting similar rates. The mean severity was 45 days' absence and the lower limb was involved in 70% of injuries, with 78% involving contact [11].

17.3.2 Youth and Junior Rugby

At the youth and academy level, injuries occur at a lower late of 47 per 1000 player hours, and the rate at school is 35 per 1000 player hours. The most common injury at this level is a ligament sprain of the lower limb. In Under-16 rugby the Injury Incidence Density (IID) of 28.8 per 1000 player hours has been reported with an injury burden of 379.2 days per 1000 h of play. The ball carrier is the most commonly affected [12].

Recurrent injuries in school rugby accounted for 5% of all injuries. Seventy eight percent of recurrences occurred within 2 months of a return to play. The injuries that provided the greatest burden were concussions, and ankle and lumbar muscle injuries [13].

In Portuguese youth rugby, injuries occurred at a rate of 138 per 1000 h of match play compared to 1.2 per 1000 h during training. With only 2 days between games the injury rate was higher than if games were played every 3 days. Injuries most commonly occurred during the third quarter of the game (44.8%) [14]. In Under-18 players in Portugal the injury rate per match was 42.85 per 1000 player hours compared to 55.8 per 1000 h play at senior level. The mean time loss per injury was 20.79 days with the lower limbs and contact events occurring at 60.5% and 65.1% [15].

In Elite English Schoolboy rugby union, those enrolled into an Achieving Academic and Sporting Excellence programme reported a greater incidence of concussion at 20 per 1000 h play rather than symptoms at sub-elite matches. In both groups greater than 50% of injuries were sustained in the tackle [16].

In youth rugby weeks in South Africa injury risk decreased with increasing age, which was thought to be related to the recognition of concussion in the age groups studied [17].

In Australian School Level Rugby Union (U-19) an overall injury rate of 23.7/1000 h was observed; for concussion this was 4.3/1000 h. Tackling was the most causative mechanism and this led to the recommendation of attempting to improve the technique during the contact phase of play.

17.3.3 Community Rugby

Performing injury surveillance in the community is challenging and it has been recommended to use terms of the rugby-specific consensus statement for injury surveillance studies. In the community an adapted report form for community rugby if medical support was not available [18]. Analysis of claims made in the New Zealand Accident compensation corporation provides a possible surveillance method for the non-elite rugby playing population. Overall 76% of claims were made for soft-tissue injuries. Ten percent of players were female however and sustained only 6% of injuries. The rates of injury were noted to rise rapidly through teenage years to the early 20s for male players and then decrease into the mid-30s. For female players the injury rate does not decrease as players move into their mid-30s [19].

The Accident Compensation Corporation data for women's community rugby revealed that the knee was the most commonly recorded site (44%) [20].

A systematic analysis and meta-analysis of injuries in amateur male rugby union have revealed an injury rate of 46.8/1000 player hours that contact events are riskier with the tackler having the greatest risk [21].

The use of a rugby-specific Web-based injury surveillance system for community data collection has been adopted in 21 out of 40 clubs in Ireland. The main barriers to data collection were considered to be player adherence (71%) and availability of medical staff (24%) [22].

When patterns of injury have been studied over time the severity of injury has been noted to be often greater in the lower levels of the game [23], suggesting that this is where prevention through regulation could have the greatest effect on injury reduction.

17.3.4 Rugby League

A prospective study of the incidence of knee injury in rugby league has shown that there are 616.7 injuries per 1000 players, with the medial collateral ligament being the most commonly injured with rates of 416.7/1000 players. The most common mechanism was being tackled and the median time to return to play was 1 day; however anterior cruciate ligament injuries accounted for the longest time to return to play of 236 days [24].

Within rugby league semi-professional players have a higher concussion risk than professional or amateur participants according to a pooled analysis. Data was extracted and pooled from 25 studies. Amateur rugby league had the highest incidence of concussion activities with 19/1000 match hours. Semi-professional league had the highest concussive injury rate with training activities of 3.1/1000 training. Semi-professionals had a three times greater concussion risk than amateur match participation. There was also nearly a 600x greater risk of concussion than professionals during training [25]. This is probably due to semi-professional training consisting of tackling and other contact drills rather than strength and conditioning training.

In an epidemiological prospective cohort study of rugby league match injuries from the European Super League using an online survey tool, 57/1000 h with an average of 34 days missed per injury were reported. The final 20 min of the game was the most significant period for injury occurrence. Forwards had the highest injury incidence and tackle activities were the commonest mechanism as in rugby league. The most common diagnoses were concussion or hamstring tears 5/1000 h and the most frequent area of injury was the knee with 10/1000 h of play [1].

The head impact exposure from match participation in a season of women's rugby league domestic competition has been studied in which 21 players wore wireless impact-measuring devices. A mean of 184 ± 18 impacts per match occurred which is 14 impacts per player. Positionally a prop had the greatest mean number of impacts with 29 impacts per match and a second row had the highest median acceleration. Forwards sustained more impacts than backs and the impacts had a greater magnitude. Most impacts were to the side of the head and were sustained during the second half of the game [26].

17.3.5 Wheelchair Rugby

Wheelchair rugby offers the opportunities of an aggressive collision sport, team membership and physical fitness to athletes that have received a spinal cord injury. This has become an increasingly popular sport with many participants from a military background.

It is beyond the scope of this booklet to cover the physiologic changes and response to exercise following spinal cord injury; however increased respiratory function with sports participation is appreciated. Wheelchair rugby is a Paralympic Games sport with 96 athletes competing in Rio in 2020. 20 injuries were reported in 16 athletes comprising 3.9% of all injuries. This resulted in an injury incidence of 14.9 (95% CI 9.6–23.1)/1000 athlete days.

There is little literature on injuries sustained during wheelchair rugby although a pilot prospective 9-month study has shown that most injuries are minor with very few injuries requiring the consultation of a physician. There was an injury rate of 0.3 per athlete per training day. Offensive players were found to have higher levels of anger and aggression than defensive players [27].

17.4 Specific Rehab and Return to Play

Rehabilitation process in sport is a team working between medical staff (team doctor, physical therapist), athletic trainer and player. A good teamwork is necessary to achieve a faster and safer return to play.

The rehabilitation programme should respect the functional steps, avoiding peaks and valley in the athlete performance.

Common to other collision and contact sports it is essential that rugby players partake in a graduated resumption of all rugby activities prior to returning to play to ensure safety and minimise the risks of repeat injury.

17.5   Specific Aspects in Different Subpopulations

Many familiar with rugby would consider it likely that the more games played, the more likely that injury occurs, but conversely injury is also common when only a few games are participated in. Less than 15 or more than 35 matches in the preceding 12 months has been shown to make players more susceptible to injury. Monthly match exposure was linearly shown to be associated with injury risk, HR 1.14 per 2 SD, 90%CI 1.08–1.2, likely harmful [28].

17.6   Prevention Strategies

Regarding the risk of severe sequelae of head and cervical spine injuries, new rules have been applied and are still evolving. Several prevention strategies have been adopted in rugby union. Altering the formation of the scrum and the commands to assemble the scrum has reduced the force of the scrum. The traditional scrum with crouch, touch, pause and engage resulted in 9 Kilonewtons (KN) of force compared to crouch, touch and set resulting in 7KN.

In France over a 10-year period of 1996–2006, a rule change and the requirement for medical certification with specific training for the front row have led to a declining incidence of catastrophic cervical spine injuries.

In school boy rugby, the introduction of pre-activity movement control exercise has led to reducing of musculoskeletal injury (RR 0.28 0.14–0.51) and concussion risk (RR 0.41 0.17–0.99).

Video analysis has been introduced to aid and allow the analysis of recognition and diagnosis of head injuries and concussions. Seventy-six percent of head injuries were found to occur during tackles, with the tackler being injured more commonly (1.4/1000 player hours) than the ball carrier (0.54/1000 player hours, RR 2.59). Backs were more commonly affected than forwards with an incidence rate ratio of 1.54 (95% CI 1.28–1.84). An upright tackler was 1.5 times more likely to receive a head injury assessment than a tackler bent at the waist. The tackler's head was more likely to be below the ball carrier's head and shoulders with an incidence rate ratio of 4.25 (95% CI 3.38–5.35).

The introduction of a tailored preventative programme for specific hip injury prevention did not reduce the number of injuries but it did reduce the severity from 936 to 468 days and the prevalence from 21% to 19%. This improved recovery time by 50 days compared with a generic programme of 259 days [29].

17.7   Equipment and Protection Considerations

Players are inspected by officials prior to each game to ensure that no hard protective devices are used. The use of "skull caps" has been shown to reduce scalp lacerations but their use does not reduce concussion rates.

The playing surfaces in other sports have anecdotally been thought to influence injury rate. In rugby however playing surface has not been shown to influence injury patterns with rates of 80 injuries per 1000 h play for artificial surfaces compared to 81.9 injuries per 1000 playing hours for grass [30].

17.8   Other Health Aspects and Diseases

As a contact sport, players are encouraged to report skin problems early and players are counselled regarding blood-borne diseases.

17.9   Match Rules with Medical Importance

Given the contact nature of rugby, lacerations are common particularly to the head. The presence of blood introduces the risk of cross infection and thereby players with bleeding must be removed from the field of play until the bleeding ceases. World Rugby permits 15 min for this process to occur during which a temporary substitute may be allowed to play. If the bleeding cannot be stopped during this time, the substitution becomes permanent.

Table 17.1 Criteria for permanent removal from play or medical room head injury assessment

Immediate and permanent removal from play or medical room assessment	Off-pitch screening tool criteria
Confirmed loss of consciousness	Head impact event where diagnosis not immediately apparent
Suspected loss of consciousness	
Tonic posturing	
Convulsion	
Balance disturbance/ataxia	Possible behavioural changes
Definite confusion	
Not orientated in time, place or person	Possible confusion
	Injury with a potential risk of concussion
Clearly dazed	
Definite behavioural changes	
Oculomotor abnormalities	Other concerning feature
Other on-field identification of sign or symptom of concussion	

Following a head injury, players will be assessed for concussion and can be removed immediately from play (IPR—Immediate and Permanent Removal) or the player may undergo a Head Injury Assessment (HIA). For this to occur a player is also permitted a temporary substitution but for 10 min. This incorporates video analysis, questions from the Standardised Concussion Assessment Tool and gait assessment. Please see the chapter on head injury/concussion assessment for specific details.

If players have sustained a head laceration and a head injury, the wound must be sutured and a head injury assessment completed within 15 min. In the English Premiership all teams have a medical representative watching the game on a computer lagging 5 s behind play permitting phases of play to be tagged for inspection. These can be highlighted to the doctor for review. In addition all games are watched retrospectively by an independent observer and the medical response is noted to each tackle or incident. These are discussed with the medical teams following the match (Table 17.1).

17.10 Summary

Although rugby is a contact collision sport and injuries commonly occur, the rules of the game have been adapted to make it safer. The training, medical provision and scrutiny that pitch-side medical personnel are subject to make rugby as safe a game as possible [31].

- On average a club will have 18% of players unavailable as a consequence of match injuries.
- Each club will suffer 10 knee injuries per season.
- On average, a professional rugby union player is more likely than not to sustain a concussion after 25 matches.
- Players have a 60% greater risk of time loss due to injury after concussion.

References

1. King D, Hume P, Cummins C, Pearce A, Clark T, Foskett A, Barnes M. Match and training injuries in women's rugby union: a systematic review of published studies. Sports Med. 2019;49(10):1559–74. https://doi.org/10.1007/s40279-019-01151-4.
2. Fuller JT, Thewlis D, Tsiros MD, Brown NAT, Hamill J, Buckley JD. Longer-term effects of minimalist shoes on running performance, strength and bone density: a 20-week follow-up study. Eur J Sport Sci. 2019;19(3):402–12. https://doi.org/10.1080/17461391.2018.1505958. Epub 2018 Aug 13.
3. Cosgrave M, Williams S. The epidemiology of concussion in professional rugby union in Ireland. Phys Ther Sport. 2019;35:99–105. https://doi.org/10.1016/j.ptsp.2018.11.010. Epub 2018 Nov 28.
4. Guskiewicz KM, Weaver NL, Padua DA, Garrett WE Jr. Epidemiology of concussion in collegiate and high school football players. Am J Sports Med. 2000;28(5):643–50. https://doi.org/10.1177/03635465000280050401.
5. Zemper ED, Tate DG, Roller S, Forchheimer M, Chiodo A, Nelson VS, Scelza W. Assessment of a holistic wellness program for persons with spinal cord injury. Am J Phys Med Rehabil. 2003;82(12):957–68; quiz 969–71. https://doi.org/10.1097/01.PHM.0000098504.78524.E2.
6. Shuttleworth-Rdwards AB, Radloff SE. Compromised visuomotor processing speed in players of Rugby Union from school through to the national adult level. Arch Clin Neuropsychol. 2008;23(5):511–20. https://doi.org/10.1016/j.acn.2008.05.002. Epub 2008 Jun 27.
7. Cunningham J, Broglio S, Wilson F. Influence of playing rugby on long-term brain health following retirement: a systematic review and narrative synthesis. BMJ Open Sport Exerc Med. 2018;4(1):e000356. https://doi.org/10.1136/bmjsem-2018-000356.
8. Gouttebarge V, Hopley P, Kerkhoffs G, Verhagen E, Viljoen W, Wylleman P, Lambert M. A 12-month prospective cohort study of symptoms of common mental disorders among professional rugby players. Eur J Sport Sci. 2018;18(7):1004–12. https://doi.org/10.1080/17461391.2018.1466914. Epub 2018 Apr 26.
9. Badenhorst M, Verhagen EALM, van Mechelen W, Lambert MI, Viljoen W, Readhead C, Baerecke G, Brown JC. A comparison of catastrophic

injury incidence rates by Provincial Rugby Union in South Africa. J Sci Med Sport. 2017;20(7):643–47. https://doi.org/10.1016/j.jsams.2017.01.232. Epub 2017 Jan 24.

10. Cruz-Ferreira AM, Cruz-Ferreira EM, Silva JD, Ferreira RM, Santiago LM, Taborda-Barata L. Epidemiology of injuries in Portuguese senior male rugby union sevens: a cohort prospective study. Phys Sportsmed. 2018;46(2):255–61. https://doi.org/10.10 80/00913847.2018.1441581. Epub 2018 Feb 27.

11. Fuller CW, Taylor A, Molloy MG. Epidemiological study of injuries in international Rugby Sevens. Clin J Sport Med. 2010;20(3):179–84. https://doi. org/10.1097/JSM.0b013e3181df1eea.

12. Sewry N, Verhagen E, Lambert M, van Mechelen W, Readhead C, Viljoen W, Brown J. Seasonal time-loss match injury rates and burden in South African under-16 rugby teams. J Sci Med Sport. 2019;22(1):54–8. https://doi.org/10.1016/j.jsams.2018.06.007. Epub 2018 Jun 19.

13. Archbold HAP, Rankin AT, Webb M, Nicholas R, Eames NWA, Wilson RK, Henderson LA, Heyes GJ, Davies R, Bleakley CM. Recurrent injury patterns in adolescent rugby. Phys Ther Sport. 2018;33:12–7. https://doi.org/10.1016/j.ptsp.2018.06.005. Epub 2018 Jun 18.

14. Solis-Mencia C, Ramos-Álvarez JJ, Murias-Lozano R, Aramberri M, Saló JC. Epidemiology of injuries sustained by elite under-18 rugby players. J Athl Train. 2019;54(11):1187–91. https://doi.org/10.4085/1062-6050-510-18.

15. Cruz-Ferreira AM, Cruz-Ferreira EM, Ribeiro PB, Santiago LM, Taborda-Barata L. Epidemiology of time-loss injuries in senior and under-18 Portuguese male rugby players. J Hum Kinet. 2018;62:73–80. https://doi.org/10.1515/hukin-2017-0159.

16. Barden C, Stokes K. Epidemiology of injury in elite english schoolboy rugby union: a 3-year study comparing different competitions. J Athl Train. 2018;53(5):514–20. https://doi.org/10.4085/1062-6050-311-16. Epub 2018 Jun 7.

17. Sewry N, Verhagen E, Lambert M, van Mechelen W, Marsh J, Readhead C, Viljoen W, Brown J. Trends in time-loss injuries during the 2011–2016 South African rugby youth weeks. Scand J Med Sci Sports. 2018;28(9):2066–73. https://doi.org/10.1111/sms.13087. Epub 2018 Apr 10.

18. Brown JC, Cross M, England M, Finch CF, Fuller GW, Kemp SPT, Quarrie K, Raftery M, Stokes K, Tucker R, Verhagen E, Fuller CW. Guidelines for community-based injury surveillance in rugby union. J Sci Med Sport. 2019;22(12):1314–8. https://doi.org/10.1016/j.jsams.2019.08.006. Epub 2019 Aug 12.

19. Quarrie K, Gianotti S, Murphy I. Correction to: injury risk in New Zealand rugby union: a nationwide study of injury insurance claims from 2005 to 2017. Sports Med. 2020;50(2):429. https://doi.org/10.1007/s40279-019-01202-w.

20. King D, Hume PA, Hardaker N, Cummins C, Clark T, Pearce AJ, Gissane C. Female rugby union injuries in New Zealand: a review of five years (2013–2017) of accident compensation corporation moderate to severe claims and costs. J Sci Med Sport. 2019;22(5):532–7. https://doi.org/10.1016/j.jsams.2018.10.015. Epub 2018 Nov 6.

21. Yeomans C, Kenny IC, Cahalan R, Warrington GD, Harrison AJ, Hayes K, Lyons M, Campbell MJ, Comyns TM. The incidence of injury in amateur male rugby union: a systematic review and meta-analysis. Sports Med. 2018;48(4):837–48. https://doi.org/10.1007/s40279-017-0838-4.

22. Yeomans C, Comyns TM, Cahalan R, Hayes K, Costello V, Warrington GD, Harrison AJ, Lyons M, Campbell MJ, Glynn LG, Kenny IC. The relationship between physical and wellness measures and injury in amateur rugby union players. Phys Ther Sport. 2019;40:59–65. https://doi.org/10.1016/j.ptsp.2019.08.012. Epub 2019 Aug 31.

23. Viviers PL, Viljoen JT, Derman W. A review of a decade of rugby union injury epidemiology: 2007–2017. Sports Health. 2018;10(3):223–7. https://doi.org/10.1177/1941738118757178. Epub 2018 Feb 14.

24. Awwad GEH, Coleman JH, Dunkley CJ, Dewar DC. An analysis of knee injuries in rugby league: the experience at the newcastle knights professional rugby league team. Sports Med Open. 2019;5(1):33. https://doi.org/10.1186/s40798-019-0206-z.

25. King D, Hume P, Gissane C, Clark T. Semi-Professional rugby league players have higher concussion risk than professional or amateur participants: a pooled analysis. Sports Med. 2017;47(2):197–205. https://doi.org/10.1007/s40279-016-0576-z.

26. King DA, Hume PA, Gissane C, Kieser DC, Clark TN. Head impact exposure from match participation in women's rugby league over one season of domestic competition. J Sci Med Sport. 2018;21(2):139–46. https://doi.org/10.1016/j.jsams.2017.10.026. Epub 2017 Oct 28.

27. Bauerfeind J, Koper M, Wieczorek J, Urbański P, Tasiemski T. Sports injuries in wheelchair rugby - a pilot study. J Hum Kinet. 2015;48:123–32. https://doi.org/10.1515/hukin-2015-0098.

28. Williams S, Trewartha G, Kemp SPT, Brooks JHM, Fuller CW, Taylor AE, Cross MJ, Shaddick G, Stokes KA. How much rugby is too much? a seven-season prospective cohort study of match exposure and injury risk in professional rugby union players. Sports Med. 2017;47(11):2395–402. https://doi.org/10.1007/s40279-017-0721-3.

29. Evans KL, Hughes J, Williams MD. Reduced severity of lumbo-pelvic-hip injuries in professional rugby union players following tailored preventative programmes. J Sci Med Sport. 2018;21(3):274–79. https://doi.org/10.1016/j.jsams.2017.07.004. Epub 2017 Jul 12.

30. Ranson C, George J, Rafferty J, Miles J, Moore I. Playing surface and UK professional rugby union injury risk. J Sports Sci. 2018;36(21):2393–8. https://doi.org/10.1080/02640414.2018.1458588. Epub 2018 Mar 29.

31. Carmont MR, Kelberine F, Lester C. Rugby. In: Krutsch W, Mayr HO, Musahl V, Della Villa F, Tscholl PM, Jones H. (eds) Injury and health risk management in sports. Springer, Berlin, Heidelberg. 2020. https://doi.org/10.1007/978-3-662-60752-7_73.

Skiing

18

Diego García-Germán, Gonzalo Samitier, and Hubert Hörterer

18.1 Introduction

Skiing and other snow sports activities are enjoyed worldwide. Accessibility is increasing with expansion of ski areas, better ski lifts, and the use of snow machines. The Winter Olympics being held in Asian countries has expanded skiing globally. Skiing is performed in nature, subjected to climate changes and a cold environment. It is a physical activity with a risk of injury as speed and falling are part of the sport. Several risk factors are associated with accidents such as crowded resorts, lack of risk awareness at high speeds, and technically challenging maneuvers.

Alpine skiing implies a risk of injury. Risk of dying is very low, but risk of sustaining an anterior cruciate ligament (ACL) injury is 365 times higher than that of the general population, being similar to American Football (30–70 injuries per 100,000 skiers per day) [1]. Injury incidence has not changed significantly over time [2].

18.2 Injury Distribution

The distribution of skiing injuries has been extensively studied. Most series find a predominance of lower extremity injuries as opposed to snowboarding where upper extremity injuries are more frequent [3, 4]. ACL injury is the most frequent diagnosis in most series [5].

Injury incidence could be similar between sexes, as opposed to other sports. ACL injury incidence is similar in men and women in the World Cup [6], with a slight higher incidence in women in their late teens [7]. A genetic predisposition to injury could be present in ACL injuries with affected skiers having a higher risk of having parents with ACL tears [8].

Injury pattern could be different in adult and adolescent skiers. The prevalence of shoulder and knee injuries is higher in adults than in children. In contrast, the prevalence of skiing lower leg fractures is higher in children than in adults. More children than adult alpine skiers suffer their injury in terrain parks [9].

In the hand, ulnar collateral ligament "skier thumb" injuries can account for up to 80% of all upper extremity injuries in skiers [10].

D. García-Germán (✉)
Orthopedic Surgeon, Clínica DKF, Madrid, Spain

Royal Spanish Winter Sports Federation, Madrid, Spain

G. Samitier
Royal Spanish Winter Sports Federation, Madrid, Spain

Centro Médico Quirosalud Aribau, Barcelona, Spain

H. Hörterer
Medical Committee, International Ski Federation FIS, Oberhofen, Switzerland

FIS Injury and Prevention Programm ISPP, Rottach-Egern, Germany
e-mail: mail@dr-hubert-hoerterer.de

© The Author(s), under exclusive license to Springer-Verlag GmbH, DE, part of Springer Nature 2022
G. L. Canata, H. Jones (eds.), *Epidemiology of Injuries in Sports*,
https://doi.org/10.1007/978-3-662-64532-1_18

18.3   Serious Injuries in Skiing

The risk of traumatic death while skiing has not changed over the past 30 years [11]: 0.71 deaths per million event days of exposure. The risk of death expressed as the number of fatalities per million hours of exposure seems to be on the same order of magnitude as death by car or bicycle, in the range of approximately 0.1 deaths per million hours of exposure. Data from 22 fatalities occurred while skiing shows that the main cause is craniocerebral and chest trauma [12].

Head injury is the most frequent reason for hospital admission [13] and the most common cause of death among skiers and snowboarders, with an 8% fatality rate among those admitted to hospital with head injuries [14]. Freestyle skiers have a twofold risk of sustaining a head injury compared to alpine skiers [15].

Helmets are mandatory for competitive skiers in the Iternational Ski Federation (FIS) World Cup events in all disciplines. In contrast, ski resorts do not typically require helmet use. The use of helmets has increased among recreational skiers and snowboarders [16], and their use is higher among children [17].

Opponents of mandatory helmet use even claim that helmets may increase the risk because they may lead to a reduced field of vision, impaired hearing, or increased speed through a false feeling of security and thus increase the incidence of collisions, which are the cause of many severe injuries [17].

Using a helmet was associated with a 60% reduction in the risk for head injury when comparing skiers with head injuries with uninjured controls [18]. Helmet use has increased from 6% in 1996 to 84% in 2013 [19].

The most frequent among these was traumatic brain injury, followed by spinal injuries [20]. Spinal injuries frequently occur in combination with other body regions. While the overall injury rate seen with skiing and snowboarding has decreased, the rate of spinal injuries has plateaued or slightly increased. The most frequently observed spinal injuries among skiers and snowboarders are vertebral fractures [21]. Less than 1% of sports-related spinal cord injuries fully recover by hospital discharge. Reported fatality rates for skiing and snowboarding injuries range from 0.8 to 3% [22].

Death of cardiac origin should be considered in older skiers presenting risk factors, and therefore proper previous work-up is recommended in these skiers [23]. Avalanches should be considered when back country skiing, where asphyxia is the main cause of death (75%) followed by trauma [24].

18.4   Equipment-Related Factors

Improvement in the ski boot-binding interface in the 1960s and 1970s included high plastic boots as opposed to low leather boots and self-releasing bindings. This change drastically reduced the incidence of ankle injuries in skiing with an important increase in knee injuries [24].

Ski geometry has been related to injury incidence. So called "carving" skis introduced to market in the 1990s have become the mainstay in the ski industry. The higher side cut and lower turn radius allows easier turns with less slippage or drag and more speed. Being more reactive and having less energy dissipation these types of skis could increase the injury incidence, as was apparent after the introduction in the World Cup. In the 2012/2013 season, FIS changed the regulation on ski geometry including longer skis with less side cut and higher turn radius. Following these changes, injury incidence decreased in upper extremity and minor injuries, but ACL injury incidence was not changed [25]. In the 2017/2018 season, FIS changed regulations again allowing bigger side cut and lower turn radius (Fig. 18.1).

In younger skiers, equipment could have a high impact on injury incidence. Poor boot fit is a major factor leading to lower leg fractures and sprains, especially among children [26, 27]. If the foot can easily move within the boot, then the binding release function is compromised. Children have a greater risk of these injuries and therefore need the best-fitting equipment [28].

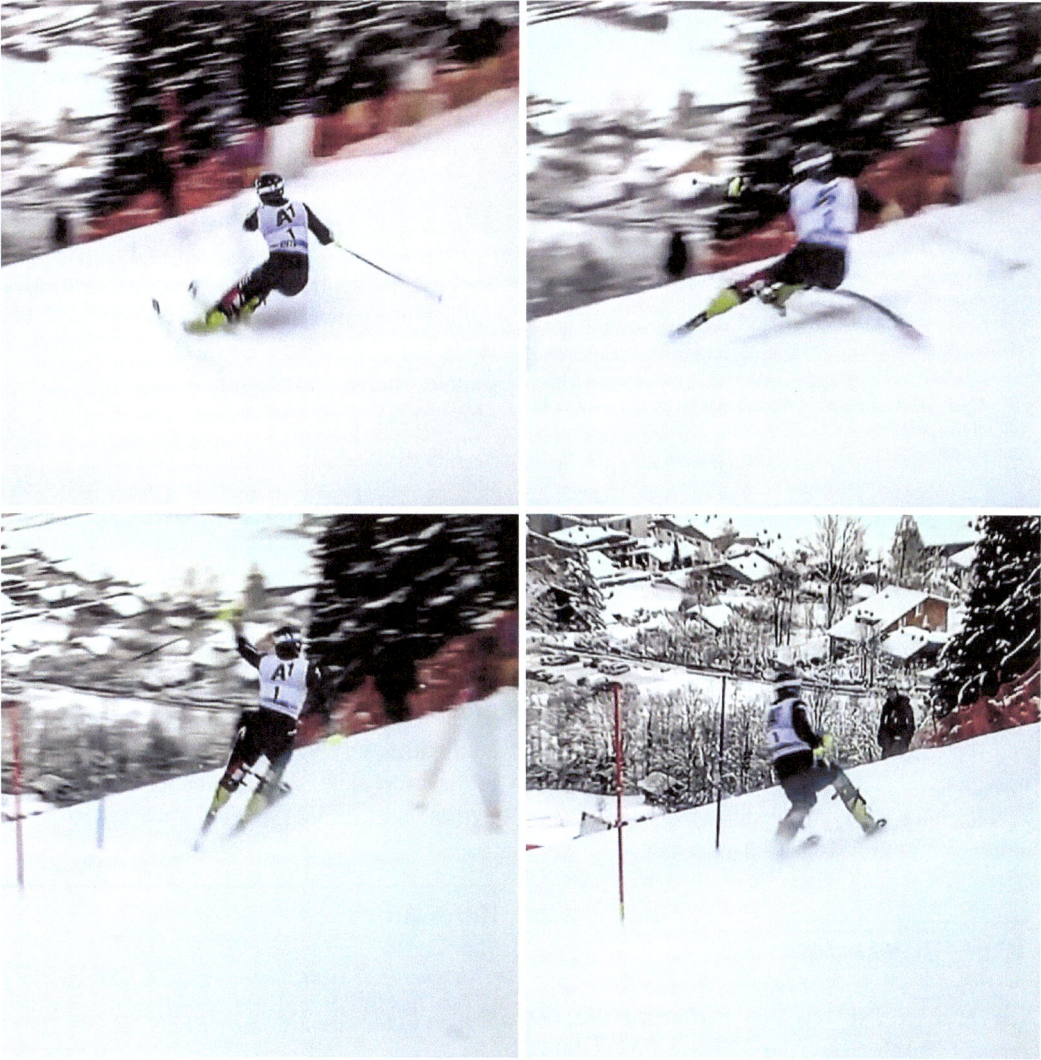

Fig. 18.1 Typical "slip-catch" ACL injury mechanism in alpine skiing, including sudden internal rotation of the knee

18.5 Competitive Versus Recreational Skiing

In 2006, the FIS together with Oslo Trauma Research Center began an injury surveillance system (ISS) [3]. Anterior cruciate ligament injury mechanisms have been well described and documented in competitive alpine skiing by means of video analysis [6].

Injury incidence is 36.7/100 skiers per season. It increases from Slalom 4.9/1000 runs) to Downhill (17.2/1000 runs). If adjusted to exposure time, related to length of the run, these incidences are similar [1]. Injury incidence is higher during race runs (45%) compared to training runs (25%). This difference could be higher if the number of race runs is compared to training runs during the season [29].

Knee injuries are the most frequent, representing 35.6% of all injuries in FIS Ski World Cup. ACL injury is the most frequent diagnosis representing 13.6% of all injuries [3] and 50% of knee injuries [29]. Most knee injuries are not related to fall but to indirect injury to the knee as a result of sudden internal rotation of the knee.

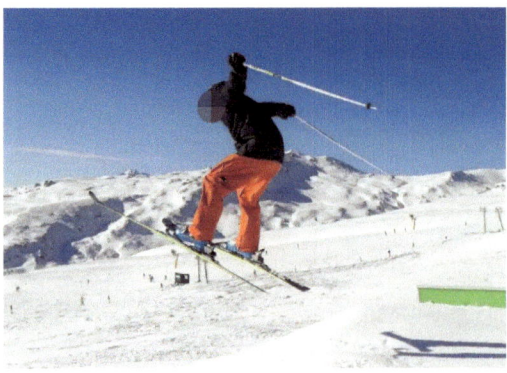

Fig. 18.2 ACL injury in recreational skiers could be related to jumps

Pujol et al. found a 28% prevalence of ACL injury in competitive elite alpine skiers with a 19% of re-ruptures and 30% of contra lateral ACL tears [2].

The main mechanisms are slip–catch, landing back-weighted, and dynamic snowplough. Differences between competitive alpine skiing and recreational skiing are obvious. Jumps and non-jump related to landing back-weighted could be the main injury mechanisms in recreational alpine skiing [30] (Fig. 18.2).

18.6   Risk Factors

The retrospective analysis performed did not reveal a link between the physical fitness of an athlete and the incidence of ACL injury. Generally, it remains questionable to what extend fitness tests can be related to injury prediction with sufficient accuracy [31]. A slight decrease in incidence of ACL injury has been found with higher "core" strength [7].

Multiple risk factors have been related to snow quality and weather. Cold temperatures have a relation with injury incidence and competition is limited to temperatures above −24°. Bad visibility has been found to increase injuries [32].

Similar to other sports, the type of surface where practice occurs has an influence on injury incidence. Not only jumps, bumps, or other features can have an effect but also the quality of snow itself can raise the reactivity and ground reaction forces transmitted to the knees and

increase injuries [33]. Harder and icier snow will give place to more slip and energy dissipation lowering the risk of "slip–catch" mechanism in ACL injuries [4].

18.7   Prevention Strategies

Specific prevention strategies have proven to reduce injury incidence in other sports [34]. One study showed a decrease in injury incidence in trained skiing professionals working at ski resorts [24].

The use of knee braces has been debated. It is unclear if it has a role in primary prevention of ACL injury. Some studies have proven a decrease in ACL re-rupture after reconstruction and less giving-way episodes in ACL deficient skiers [35, 36].

Unfortunately, injury is inherently related to skiing. ACL injury incidence has not changed significantly throughout the years. It is important to know the epidemiology and risk factors associated with injury in skiing. Future actions should be taken to make skiing safer for both competitive and recreational skiers.

References

1. Engebretsen L, Steffen K, Alonso JM. Sports injuries and illnesses during the Winter Olympic Games 2010. Br J Sports Med. 2010;44:772–80.
2. Pujol N, Blanchi MP, Chambat P. The incidence of anterior cruciate ligament injuries among competitive Alpine skiers: a 25-year investigation. Am J Sports Med. 2007;35:1070–4.
3. Florenes TW, Nordsletten L, Heir S, Bahr R. Recording injuries among World Cup skiers and snowboarders: a methodological study. Scand J Med Sci Sports. 2011;21:196–205.
4. Spörri J, Kröll J, Blake O, Amesberger G, Müller E. A qualitative approach to determine key injury risk factors in alpine ski racing. Internationaler Skiverband (FIS). 2010.
5. Kim S, Endres NK, Johnson RJ. Snowboard injuries. Trends over time and comparisons with apine skiing injuries. Am J Sports Med. 2012;40:770–6.
6. Bere T, Flørenes TW, Krosshaug T, Haugen P, Svandal I, Nordsletten L, Bahr R. A systematic video analysis of 69 injury cases in World Cup alpine skiing. Scand J Med Sci Sports. 2014;24:667–77.
7. Raschner C, Platzer HP, Patterson C, Werner I, Huber R, Hildebrandt C. The relationship between ACL injuries and physical fitness in young competitive ski

racers: a 10-year longitudinal study. Br J Sports Med. 2012;46:1065–71.

8. Westin M, Reeds-Lundqvist S, Werner S. The correlation between anterior cruciate ligament injury in elite alpine skiers and their parents. Knee Surg Sports Traumatol Arthrosc. 2016;24:697–701.

9. Ekeland A, Rødven A, Heir S. Injuries among children and adults in alpine skiing and snowboarding. J Sci Med Sport. 2019;22(Suppl 1):S3–6.

10. Van Dommelen BA, Zvirbulis RA. Upperextremity injuries in snow skiers. Am J Sports Med. 1989;17(6):751–3.

11. Shealy JE, Ettlinger CF, Johnson RJ. On-piste fatalities in recreational snow sports in the U.S. In: Johnson RJ, Shealy JE, Yamagishi T, editors. Skiing trauma and safety: sixteenth volume (ASTM STP 1474). West Conshohocken, PA: ASTM International; 2006. p. 27–4.

12. Kunz SN, Keller T, Grove C, Lochner S, Monticelli F. Fatal skiing accidents: a forensic analysis taking the example of Salzburg. Arch Kriminol. 2015;235(1–2):1–10.

13. Furrer M, Erhart S, Frutiger A, Bereiter H, Leutenegger A, Ruedi T. Severe skiing injuries: a retro- spective analysis of 361 patients including mecha- nism of trauma, severity of injury, and mortality. J Trauma. 1995;39:737–41.

14. Hackam DJ, Kreller M, Pearl RH. Snow-related recreational injuries in children: assessment of morbidity and management strategies. J Pediatr Surg. 1999;34:65–8.

15. Steenstrup SE, Bere T, Bahr R. Head injuries among FIS World Cup alpine and freestyle skiers and snowboarders: a 7-year cohort study. Br J Sports Med. 2014;48(1):41–5.

16. Macnab AJ, Smith T, Gagnon FA, Macnab M. Effect of helmet wear on the incidence of head/face and cervical spine injuries in young skiers and snowboarders. Inj Prev. 2002;8:324–7.

17. Levy AS, Smith RH. Neurologic injuries in skiers and snowboarders. Semin Neurol. 2000;20:233–45.

18. Sulheim S, Holme I, Elkeland A, Bahr R. Helmet use and risk of head injuries in alpine skiers and snowboarders. AMA. 2006;295:919–24.

19. Patrick E, Cooper JG, Daniels J. Changes in skiing and snowboardinginjury epidemiology and attitudesto safety in Big Sky, Montana, USAA Comparison of 2 Cross-sectional Studiesin 1996 and 2013. Orthop J Sports Med. 2015;3:1–6.

20. Corra S, Girardi P, De Giorgi F, Braggion M. Severe and polytraumaticinjuries among recreational skiers and snowboarders: incidence,demographics and injury patterns in South Tyrol. Eur J Emerg Med. 2012;19(2):69–72.

21. Kary JM. Acute spine injuries in skiers and snowboarders. Curr Sports MedRep. 2008;7(1):35–8.

22. De Roulet A, Inaba K, Strumwasser A, Chouliaras K, Lam L, Benjamin E, Grabo D, Demetriades D. Severe injuries associated with skiing andsnowboarding: a national trauma data bank study. J Trauma Acute Care Surg. 2017;82(4):781–6.

23. Burtscher M. Risk and protective factors for sudden cardiac death during leisure activities in the mountains: an update. Heart Lung Cir. 2017;26:757–62.

24. Ettlinger CF, Johnson RJ, Shealy J. A method to help reduce the risk of serious knee sprains incurred in alpine skiing. Am J Sports Med. 1996;23:531–7.

25. Haaland B, Steenstrup SE, Bere T, Roald Bahr R, Nordsletten L. Injury rate and injury patterns in FIS World Cup Alpine skiing (2006–2015): have the new ski regulations made an impact? Br J Sports Med. 2016;1:32–6.

26. Deibert MC, Aronsson DD, Johnson RJ, Ettlinger CF, Shealy JE. Skiing injuries in children, adolescents and adults. J Bone Joint Surg Am. 1998;80(1):25–32.

27. Ettlinger CF, Johnson RJ, Shealy JE. Functional release characteristics of alpine ski equipment. In: Johnson RJ, Shealy JE, Yamagishi T, editors. Skiing trauma and safety: sixteenth international symposium (ASTM STP 1474). West Conshohocken, PA: ASTM International; 2006. p. 65–74.

28. Johnson RJ, Ettlinger CF, Shealy JE. Myths concerning alpine skiing injuries. Sports Health. 2009;1:486–92.

29. Stevenson H, Webster J, Johnson RJ, Beynnon BD. Gender differences in knee injury epidemiology among competitive alpine ski racers. Iowa Orthop J. 1998;18:64–6.

30. Vázquez S, Cristina Ávila C, Virginia Herrero V, García-Germán D. Anterior cruciate ligament injury mechanisms in recreational skiing, are they different from competitive alpine skiing? Poster. ESSKA Specialty Days Meeting. Madrid; 2019.

31. Schmitt KU, Hörterer N, Vogt M, Frey WO, Lorenzetti S. Investigating physical fitness and race performance as determinants for the ACL injury risk in Alpine ski racing. Sports Sci Med Rehabil. 2016;8:23.

32. Jordan MJ, Aagaard P, Herzog W. Anterior cruciate ligament injury/reinjury in alpine ski racing: a narrative review. Open Acc J Sports Med. 2017;8: 71–83.

33. Fauve M, Rhyner HU, Schneebeli M. Preparation and maintenance of pistes. Handbook for practitioners. Davos: Swiss Federal Institute for Snow and Avalanche Research; 2002.

34. Zebis MK, Andersen LL, Brandt M, Bandholm T, Thorborg K, Hölmich P, Aagaard P, et al. Effects of evidence-based prevention training on neuromuscular and biomechanical risk factors for ACL injury in adolescent female athletes: a randomized controlled trial. Br J Sports Med. 2016;50:552–7.

35. Jordan MJ, Aagaard P, Herzog W. Rapid hamstrings/quadriceps strength in ACL-reconstructed elite alpine ski racers. Med Sci Sports Exerc. 2015;47:109–19.

36. Kocher MS, Sterett WI, Briggs KK, Zurakowski D, Steadman JR. Effect of functional bracing on subsequent knee injury in ACL-deficient professional skiers. J Knee Surg. 2003;16:87–92.

Alpine Skiing

19

Amelie Stoehr and Hermann Mayr

19.1 Characteristics of the Sport

Skiing has a long history of more than 5000 years. Primarily, it has been used for transport but nowadays has more recreational and sports value. Alpine or downhill skiing was developed around the 1930s with the invention of ski lifts. A relevant characteristic is fixed-heel bindings that attach at both toe and heel of the skier's boot. Alpine skiing became an Olympic sport at the 1936 Winter Games in Garmisch-Partenkirchen, Germany. There are the following disciplines in Alpine ski racing that vary in duration, number of changes in direction, course, terrain, and jumps:

1. Super G and Downhill: Speed events.
2. Giant Slalom and Slalom: Technical events.
3. Alpine Combined: Combination of Downhill and Slalom event.

A. Stoehr (✉)
OCM Clinic Munich, Munich, Germany

H. Mayr
Department of Orthopedic and Trauma Surgery,
Albert Ludwig University of Freiburg,
Freiburg, Germany

19.2 Physiological and Biomechanical Demands on Athletes

Important refinements in preparation of slopes, design of courses, technical equipment, and the skills of professional alpine skiers have all contributed to the present significance of Alpine skiing. A more direct interaction between athlete and snow has developed by improved snow preparation with harder surfaces and better equipment (Fig. 19.1).

Racing courses today are more challenging with greater ground reaction forces. Athletes needed to adapt their training methods to meet these new demands [1]. Owing to the extremely high variability of external conditions, the technique involved is similar to open motor skill sports. Variations in snow conditions, speed, course setting, terrain, and visibility all put high demands on the athlete. In competition, an athlete must adapt to any unexpected changes that may occur since the course has been inspected. Alpine ski racing is a challenging sport for an athlete's physical capacities, including power, strength, aerobic and anaerobic capacity, coordination and motor control, balance, and mobility. Nowadays, higher bone and muscle mass promotes downhill performance. Slalom skiers seem to be leaner, whereas downhill racers are the heaviest. Leg strength has been shown to corre-

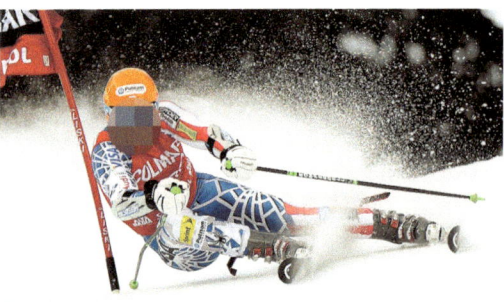

Fig. 19.1 Typical situation of an Alpine ski racer

Table 19.1 Injuries recorded from 2006–2019 by FIS ISS in Ski athletes ($n = 1322$)

Injured body regions	Percentage in %
Knee	41.3
Back and pelvis	9.2
Shoulders	6.1
Hands and fingers	9.7
Lower leg and Achilles tendon	9.0
Head and face	9.4

Table 19.2 Types of ACL injury mechanisms in skiers

Competitive skiing	Recreational skiing
Slip–catch	Boot-induced anterior drawer
Landing back-weighted	Phantom foot
Dynamic snow plough	

late highly with performance in the downhill and giant slalom events [2].

19.3 Epidemiology of Injuries

There are relevant internal and external risk factors for Alpine skiing injuries [3]. Internal factors affect the risk of sustaining an injury such as age, sex, biomechanics, technical skills, fatigue, conditioning, previous injuries, and risk-taking behavior, whereas external factors such as equipment, snow conditions, weather, and course setting may also have an influence. Usually, a complex interaction between a sudden unexpected event and possible risk factors results in the injury. Since the introduction of fixed shell ski boots in the 1960s/70s, the knee joint is predominantly exposed in terms of overloads and injuries. Approximately 42,000 injuries are registered in the Alps every year for recreational skiing. In the season 2016/2017, the mainly injured body parts were the knee with 31.6%, the shoulder with 22.2%, the head with 11%, the back with 9.4%, and the hip and pelvis with 9.1%. Women had almost double the risk to sustain a knee injury than men in recreational skiing [4]. An initiative was taken by FIS (International Ski Federation) to establish an injury surveillance system (the FIS ISS) prior to the 2006/07 winter season to be able to monitor injury risk and injury pattern in the Alpine Skiing World Cup over time (Table 19.1).

Most of the injuries to the head and upper body resulted from crashes, while the majority of knee injuries occurred while skiing and turning. Gate contact resulted in 30% of all injuries, while only 9% happen at contact with safety nets; 46% of all injuries arose in the final section of the course. In competitive skiing, men had a significantly higher risk of injury, with the knee being responsible for 60% of absences longer than 6 weeks; 50% of those athletes sustained an anterior cruciate ligament (ACL) tear. When racing downhill, the skier must resist large centrifugal forces at a high speed while squatting and holding the knees in a position that places the ACL at risk of injury. Three main types of ACL injury mechanisms in competitive skiing were identified (Table 19.2) [5].

The "slip catch" mechanism is described by loss of pressure on the outer ski and while extending the outer knee to regain contact, the inside edge of the outer ski catches the snow abruptly, forcing the knee into internal rotation and valgus loading. A similar loading pattern was recognized for the "dynamic snowplough." The third injury mechanism, "the landing back-weighted" is described as the skier being out of balance backward after jumping and landing on the ski tails on extended knees. The loading mechanism is suggested to be a combination of boot-induced anterior drawer, knee joint compression, and quadriceps anterior drawer. For recreational skiers, two typical injury mechanisms are known (Table 19.2). When the boot-induced anterior drawer pushes the lower leg forward while fixed in the ski boot, the phantom foot experiences internal rotation stress and deep knee flexion, whereby the ski acts as a lever and allows the lower leg to be twisted in relation to the thigh.

During alpine skiing, the knee extensors have a dominant role with patella overload, patellar tendinitis, Sinding–Larsen–Johansson syndrome (inflammatory reaction of the patellar tendon origin at the tip of the patella, occasionally with osteonecrosis, "jumper's knee"), and Osgood–Schlatter disease (aseptic osteonecrosis of the tibial tuberosity). There is evidence that intensive physical strain, as in skiing, is associated with pathological changes to the growing spine. Lower back pain often occurs in ski racers through the constant impact and pressure movements in Alpine skiing. Especially in technical disciplines, the incidence seems to be higher. A ski boot bruise occurs when falling forward or back, while there is considerable stress on the upper edge of the ski boot. A so-called ski thumb is the crack of the inside ("ulnar") sideband at the base of the thumb. If a fall occurs while skiing, with the thumb stuck in the loop of the ski pole, this is forcibly bent over to the outside and behind. The result is a rupture of the lateral ligament with a lateral instability, sometimes in addition with a tear of the flexor-side joint capsule. Skull bruising, shoulder dislocation, fractures of the thigh, collarbone, and ankle are also common injuries when skiing.

19.4 Rehabilitation and Return to Play

Skiers undergoing ACL reconstruction surgery may suffer from a second injury to the same knee or even an ACL injury in the uninjured knee. A ski rehabilitation program should emphasize slow eccentric loading and strength as well as endurance [6]. From a biology standpoint, the ACL needs to "remodel," or grow new blood vessels after it is replaced. This takes about 9 months. However, the new ACL may be less than half of its original strength from 8–12 months after surgery. Therefore, in the early rehabilitation phase after ACL reconstruction, protecting the healing tissue, increasing joint mobility, and normalizing gait are the goals. In addition, training the rest of the body to prevent deconditioning is important. An emphasis on strong isometric recruitment of the quadriceps muscles is recommended. After the first phase, functional rehabilitation starts and can be divided into three phases: advanced rehabilitation, sport-specific training, and return-to-sport training. Details are presented in Table 19.3.

Excessive dynamic valgus loading of the knee joint is an important risk factor leading to ACL injuries. Increased hip adduction and femur internal rotation, and decreased hip extensor, abduction, and external rotation strength, are factors shown to increase dynamic valgus. Plyometric and neuromuscular stabilization exercises enable the patient to control and reduce valgus kinematics during double- and single-leg drop landing.

Several functional test batteries have been described in literature.

Prior to completion of the sport-specific phase of rehabilitation, the referring surgeon will examine the knee.

Once the athlete passes the functional sports tests with an acceptable score, the rehabilitation team releases the athlete to dry-land training with the team. The rehabilitation team coordinates with coaches and trainers to reintroduce more demanding exercises in strength and agility. At the sixth to ninth postoperative month, the athlete may return to alpine skiing, but not on a competitive-level intensity. The athlete is progressed step by step toward the requirements of their discipline. Jumps should not be performed within the first year of rehabilitation. Special case-by-case considerations are made for athletes who are required to jump, e.g., in downhill events.

Additionally, a custom made functional knee brace can be fitted after thigh girth has returned and is recommended for the first year of recovery during training and skiing [5].

The ability of rehabilitative bracing to protect the integrity of the graft has been shown in several prospective randomized controlled trials. In addition, a brace can offer neuromuscular and proprioceptive benefits.

Table 19.3 Rehabilitation after ACL reconstruction

	Goals	Minimum criteria
Early phase (weeks 1–4)	• Protection of healing tissue • Increase of joint mobility • Normalizating gait • Prevention of deconditioning	
Functional rehabilitation		
Advanced rehabilitation (from week 4–6)	• Restore muscular strength improve cardiovascular endurance • Optimize neuromuscular control, balance, and proprioception	• Symmetrical/functional passive and active knee extension • Normal gait • Minimal joint effusion • No episodes of giving way • 90% of passive knee flexion compared to the contralateral knee
Sport-specific training (from week 8–10)	• Advanced sport-cord • Plyometric exercises • Achieve strength values equal to or greater than 85% of the quadriceps and hamstring muscles of the uninjured leg	• Symmetrical bilateral squat position at 60° of knee flexion for about 30 s • Performing a single-leg squat to 30° of knee flexion while maintaining optimal axis alignment of the knee within the weight-bearing line of the lower extremity
Return-to-sport training (from months 6–9)	• Return to alpine skiing by slowly increasing training intensity	• To successfully complete functional sports tests

19.5 Prevention Strategies

There are several important points about injury prevention in recreational Alpine skiing. A good immune system and health should be natural as well as a weather and visibility adapted skiing style. Other important facts to prepare are a good warm up, ski gymnastics, good endurance, and, if possible, weight training of the lower extremities to create a good muscular stabilization of the knee joint taking into account that the quadriceps muscle acts as an antagonist toward the ACL. Increased training of the ischiocrural or hamstring muscles has shown to reduce the risk of an ACL rupture. The quadriceps acts as a knee stabilizer and protector in high flexion angles; therefore, training should be performed in knee flexion angles over 90°. As skiing is a technomotor sport, intuitive learning strategies are favored nowadays. Learning of sport-specific movements should be the base, whereas discipline-dependent training is the key in racing sports. Special training of neuromuscular motion control has shown to have protective effects. Several structured prevention programs have been developed. Psychological factors and risk-taking also play

an important role. Training intensity must be adapted to the respective development. The coaches must recognize signs of fatigue in the athlete. Overload syndromes of the musculoskeletal system should be prevented [3].

Equipment is an important factor in preventing injuries [5]. Clothing should be adapted to the weather conditions. Today, skiing helmets are worn by nearly all skiers and are partially mandatory for children. Back protectors are standard equipment for competitive athletes and are gaining acceptance in recreational skiing. In different disciplines of competitive skiing, upper and lower extremity protectors are becoming more prevalent. Appropriate skiing goggles are important for identification of terrain and hazardous spots. Airbag systems for recreational and competitive skiing are being developed. The type of ski should match the ability of the driver. To reduce the risk of lower extremity injuries, carving skis should be used at reduced speed in beginners, as the force application in curves increases exponentially with speed. The recently developed rocker skis have shown to reduce the risk of a knee injury. Available knee braces are still not able to fully protect a skier from knee injuries and wearing comfort needs to be improved. A binding release that is sensitive to physiological factors in addition to release forces should be developed and might further help to reduce the risk of severe knee injuries in the future [3].

References

1. Neumayr G, Hoertnagl H, Pfister R, Koller A, Eibl G, Raas E. Physical and physiological factors associated with success in professional alpine skiing. Int J Sports Med. 2003;24(8):571–7.
2. Gilgien M, Reid R, Raschner C, Supej M, Holmberg HC. The training of olympic alpine ski racers. Front Physiol. 2018;21(9):1772.
3. Waibel K, Jones H, Schabbehard C, Thurner B. General training aspects in consideration of prevention in sports. In: Mayr H, Zaffagnini S, editors. Prevention of injuries and overuse in sports. Berlin, Heidelberg: Springer; 2016. p. 87–99.
4. Haaland B, Steenstrup SE, Bere T, Bahr R, Nordsletten L. Injury rate and injury patterns in FIS World Cup Alpine skiing (2006-2015): have the new ski regulations made an impact? Br J Sports Med. 2016;50(1):32–6.
5. Stoehr A, Mayr H. ESSKA sports book: part 11: aspects of different sports: special considerations for winter sports: chapter 79 alpine skiing. 2019
6. Okmeyer D, Wahoff M, Mymern M. Suggestions from the field for return-to-sport rehabilitation following anterior cruciate ligament reconstruction: alpine skiing. J Orthop Sports Phys Ther. 2012;42(4):313–25.

Cross-Country Skiing

Andrey Korolev ⓘ, Nina Magnitskaya ⓘ,
Mikhail Ryazantsev ⓘ, Alexey Afanasyev ⓘ,
Denis Gerasimov, Mikhail Burtsev,
Alexey Logvinov ⓘ, Dmitriy Ilyin ⓘ,
Zhanna Pilipson ⓘ, Pavel Kadantsev ⓘ,
Aziz Zaripov ⓘ, and Bella Gazimieva ⓘ

20.1 Characteristic of the Sport

Cross-country (XC) skiing is one of the most popular winter sports and recreational activities. From 1924, XC skiing has been contested at the Winter Olympic Games. It is one of the most demanding of the aerobic endurance sports, which involves upper and lower body work, training and competing in different terrains and weather conditions. With the evolution of the

A. Korolev · D. Ilyin · P. Kadantsev
A. Zaripov · B. Gazimieva
European Medical Center (EMC), European Clinic of Sports Traumatology and Orthopaedics (ECSTO), Moscow, Russia

Department of Traumatology and Orthopedics, Medical Institution, Peoples Friendship University of Russia (PFUR), Moscow, Russia
e-mail: akorolev@emcmos.ru; dilyin@emcmos.ru; pkadantsev@emcmos.ru; azaripov@emcmos.ru; bgazimieva@emcmos.ru

N. Magnitskaya (✉) · M. Ryazantsev
A. Afanasyev · D. Gerasimov · M. Burtsev
A. Logvinov · Z. Pilipson
European Medical Center (EMC), European Clinic of Sports Traumatology and Orthopaedics (ECSTO), Moscow, Russia
e-mail: mryazantsev@emcmos.ru; aafanasyev@emcmos.ru; dgerasimov@emcmos.ru; mburtsev@emcmos.ru; alogvinov@emcmos.ru; zhpilipson@emcmos.ru

training processes, improving the technic and development of the gear, sportsmen can reach speed close to 70 km/h and overcome downhills and uphills on inclines ranging from −20 to +20% gradients.

Cross-country skiing contains two main styles (classical and skating). Because of different terrain, sportsmen have to use a lot of sub-techniques to keep their speed: diagonal stride, double poling, double poling with a kick, and herringbone—in classical style; paddle dance, double dance, single dance, and skating without poles—in skating style. In addition, the downhill tuck position (TCK) and a variety of turn techniques (TRN) are employed with both styles to pass the turns on high speed.

More explosive techniques have been developed, such as "running diagonal" and "kangaroo" double poling [1]. During the race, sportsmen are also focused on downhill turns, where they can use the accelerating step-turn technique and increase their speed even further [2].

On 2 February 1924, the International Ski Federation (FIS) was founded, to set up the rules for all skiing disciplines in which XC skiing was included. At the moment, there are several XC disciplines in the world championship and Olympic Games: individual sprint, team sprint 5 km/10 km/15 km/17–18 km/20 km/30 km/50 km, relay 4 × 10 km/3 × 5 km/4 × 5 km, skiathlon, and

G. L. Canata, H. Jones (eds.), *Epidemiology of Injuries in Sports*,
https://doi.org/10.1007/978-3-662-64532-1_20

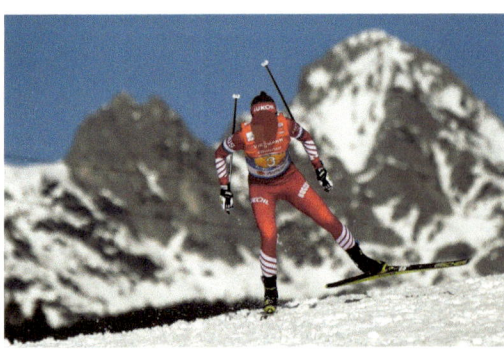

Fig. 20.1 Russian athlete during women's 4 × 5 km relay competition at the FIS Nordic World Ski Championships, 2019

marathon (Fig. 20.1). According to the 2019 FIS competition, the terrain is mandated to include approximately one-third uphill, one-third downhill, and one third flat. This requires skiers to adapt their technique according to the terrain. More than 50% of the race time is spent on the uphill sections, where the individual performance differs the most [1, 2].

Accordingly, cross-country skiing athletes design their training to improve not only their physiological capacities but also their technical and tactical expertise.

Individual performance level and physical characteristics are not the only things which affect the result. Choosing the correct sub-technique and proper gear adaptation, waxing of skis for different snow conditions and track profile play huge roles.

Previous injury and a high volume of repetitive training are two commonly reported injury risk factors in endurance athletes.

20.2 Physiological and Biomechanical Demands on Athletes

Cross-country-ski races place complex demands on athletes, with events lasting approximately 12 min to 2 h. It is one of the most demanding endurance sports, which involves protracted competitions on varying terrain employing a variety of skiing techniques that require upper and/or lower body work to different extents, often at moderate altitude and in a cold environment.

This unique discipline historically has helped researchers acquire new knowledge into the limits of human performance and regulatory capacity. There is a longstanding tradition of researchers in this field working together with coaches and athletes on training routines, monitoring progress, and refining skiing techniques improvement. This cooperation in combination with equipment progress and better track preparation, led to the significant increase in the average speed of cross-country races during the past 50 years, especially in the skating events introduced in the middle of the 1980s [2].

World-class cross-country athletes have shown some of the highest oxygen uptake (VO_{2max}) values ever reported, with values of 80–90 and 70–80 mL $\times$ kg^{-1} $\times$ min^{-1} for men and women, respectively. During competitions, temperature can be as low as −20 °C, being a serious challenge for every step of oxygen transport. Exercise ventilation rates of 250 L/min, blood volume of 9 L, cardiac outputs of >40 L/min, and stoke volumes >200 mL have all been reported among elite performers. In recent decades, demands on anaerobic capacity, upper-body power, high-speed techniques, and "tactical flexibility" have all increased for the medal contenders. The ability to efficiently transform metabolic energy into speed is a key determinant of performance for today's elite cross-country skier.

Cross-country skiing requires concentric muscle contraction with a high repetition rate, lower intensity than ski slopes, but with a much longer duration. Commonly, most of the muscles involved in the movement of the ski racer/biathlete are extensors. They provide repulsion by hands, for example, sharp extension of the shoulder (posterior deltoid muscle, latissimus dorsi, teres minor muscle, triceps), or elbow joint (triceps), as well as tremors due to extension in the lumbar spine (extensors of the trunk), extension of the thigh (gluteal muscles, muscles of the Hamstring group), extension in the knee (quadriceps) and ankle (calf, soleus muscles) joints.

The elite cross-country skier is required to master a wide range of speeds (5–70 km/h) and terrains (with inclines of −20% up to 20%). To accomplish this, they adapt the nine sub-techniques of classical skiing and skating. During a 1.5 km race, skiers change the sub-technique on average 30 times, across longer distances many hundreds of such transitions occur. Higher speeds make greater demands on producing propulsive forces to increase cycle length. Effective polling is an important strategy to enhance cycle length, which explains the popularity of more explosive techniques, such as "kangaroo" double poling and double-push skating on flat terrain. The most explosive skiers can produce double-poling forces as high as 430 N within the period of 0.05 s, as well as forces above 1600 N during the leg push-off when skating. On steep uphill, faster skiers increase cycle rate while maintaining cycle length. Over shorter sections novel techniques such as "running diagonal" and "jump skate" are used to accelerate rapidly.

There are lots of demands on modern elite cross-country skiers aspiring for medals. Terrain, with changing uphill–downhill geometry forces athletes to be tactically sharp and adaptable. The need to adapt makes them technique-aimed, through mastering more sub-techniques. Additionally, the increase of race speeds makes its demands on athlete's physiology (increasing anaerobic demands). The elite cross-country skier is an incredible human engine with possibly the best efficiency factor among all Olympic endurance sports athletes.

20.3 Epidemiology of Cross-Country Skiing

Approximately 16 million people worldwide are involved in XC, especially in Nordic countries. However, there is a lack of knowledge in the literature about the epidemiology of cross-country skiing injuries, but traditionally cross-country skiing is a sport with low risk of severe trauma. In comparison with alpine skiers, injury rate in cross-country skiers is significantly lower. According to Sochi Olympic Winter Games 2014 statistics, the injury rate among alpine skiers was 20.7% and cross-country skiers—7.7%, of which 1% were unable to come back for competition

more than 7 days. Cross-country skier injury rate varies from 2.10 injuries per 1000 exposure hours with an average age of 22.7, 2.5 injuries per 1000 exposure hours with an average age of 17–3.81 injuries per 1000 exposure hours with mean age 20.66 years [3–5].

According to published data, most cross-country skier's injuries are overuse, non-traumatic injuries. In a study by Ristolainen, the incidence for acute trauma was 0.73/1000 h and overuse—1.35/1000 h, in a study by Worth et al., the same results were published—incidence of non-traumatic injuries (2.76) and traumatic injuries (1.05).

Athletes can be injured during downhill skiing with a risk of medial collateral ligament (MCL), anterior cruciate ligament (ACL) rupture and, also, during other training events. According to Ristolainen up to 80% of injuries in XC occured during non skiing activities, in particular 35% occurred while running; according to Worth—almost three times more injuries occurred during non-training periods [3, 5]. As reported by the mentioned studies, the most typical acute traumas were ankle (25%) and lower back (17%). Extra training more than 700 h/year lead to a twice higher risk of overuse injuries and more than 5 days of training during a week lead to a five times higher risk [3]. In von Rosen et al.'s study lower extremity was also the most common (49.9%), then - lower back (15.5%), shoulder (12.1%), and hand (8.6%). In Worth et al.'s study—ankle and foot accounted for 25.6% of all injuries, and shoulder for 7.8% of all injuries. Conversely, lower back, pelvis and sacrum injuries were the most common during two World Cup seasons with an incidence rate up to 25%, shoulder and clavicle—7%, lower leg and Achilles tendon—5%. In the Ristolainen study, the most common overuse injury was the foot (22%, including toes, sole, heel and Achilles), then—knee (19%), back (17%) and shin (15%). Interestingly, overuse injuries of the back were more typical for classic technique (59%) than for skating technique. The same results were published for others overuse injuries—67% and 33%, respectively. Risk of recurrent trauma depends on previous trauma pattern, level of performance, amount of rest between championships and trainings.

Females have higher risk of injury than male, according to the studies by Ristolainen [3], von Rosen et al. [4]. and Worth et al. [5]. According to von Rosen et al., female cross-country skiers have an average weekly injury prevalence of 26.6% and substantial injury prevalence—11.1%, male—14.1%; 5.9%, respectively [4]. In Worth et al.'s study, women have almost twice a higher rate of lower extremity injury. Young skiers have a higher risk of injury in comparison with older skiers (>30 years).

20.4 Rehabilitation and Return to Play

For the most part, injuries to cross-country skiers are treated conservatively (if not concerning ruptures of ligaments or tendons).

The rehabilitation treatment of cross-country skiers, depending on the specifics of injuries (overload nature), mainly consists of:

- Reducing the sports load by up to 50% (reducing the distance to be overcome, the intensity and frequency of training, reducing the height difference in the distance),
- Temporarily replacing specific training with walking in the pool, exercise cycling and elliptical,
- Stabilization of the core muscles, tibialis anterior muscles strenthening, training of back, thigh and knee extensors,
- Training of proprioceptive skills, as well as instrumental physiotherapy (phonophoresis, electrotherapy, massage) in the acute period.

While approaching the most common cross-country ski injuries such as MCL rupture, ankle sprain, Achilles tendinitis, low back pain and medial tibial stress syndrome (MTSS), we should outline the rehabilitation principles and goals for each of them.

20.4.1 MCL

While managing MCL rupture, early functional rehabilitation includes range-of-motion and quadriceps strengthening exercises. Range-of-motion exercises are important for ligament healing. Numerous studies report that immobilization significantly diminishes ultimate load capacity of the MCL and increases osteoclastic activity at the tibial MCL insertion sites. The day after injury, the patient begins quadriceps isometric strengthening exercises, straight-leg raises, and contraction exercises of the hamstrings and quadriceps with the knee flexed and heel pressure directed toward the floor or bed. Closed kinetic chain exercises are implemented and include minisquats, toe raises, leg presses, cycling and activities with an exercise band. The bicycle seat is initially raised and gradually lowered as the patient's knee flexion improves. Once the patient achieves 90° knee flexion, passive resistance exercises for the quadriceps and hamstrings can be added.

20.4.2 Ankle Sprain

- When discussing the main rehabilitation goals after ankle sprain, the patient's top-priority program consists of full range of motion, strength and neuromuscular coordination of foot. Open-chain (OC) range of motion exercises (dorsiflexion, plantar flexion, both active and passive) and some isometrics can be performed by non-weight bearing patients as well as stretching, stationary biking and joint mobilization. While going ahead, the patient starts practicing neuromuscular and balance training as continued range of motion exercises as tolerated, constantly increasing the weight bearing from double-limbed stance to single-limb stance as well as from a firm surface to progressively more unstable, resisting perturbations, catching and throwing balls, and practicing single leg squats. The final target is gaining full muscle strength and control by adding some calf raises, resistance bands and ankle weights, jumps and jogging in a straight line. While progressing athletes should be able to perform lateral movements, change-of-direction drills and advance in more sport-specific activities using typical sport shoes.

20.4.3 Achilles

Eccentric muscle strengthening combined with ultrasound and iontophoresis procedures have proved to be effective in conservative treatment of most insertional Achilles tendon injuries. A stretching program should be added to eccentric strengthening since the majority of athletes with Achilles tendinosis have excessive pronation and limited passive dorsiflexion at the same time. In addition, orthotic devices, including heel cushions, molded ankle-foot orthoses and semirigid corrective orthotic shoe inserts, have shown the ability to improve comfort and correct over-pronation.

20.4.4 Lower Back Pain

Lower limb exercise therapy, comprising resistance training exercises such as hip abductors strengthening, hip extensors strengthening, leg press, single-leg squat, and wall-sit exercises has shown to be a promising approach to the clinical management of nonspecific chronic lower back pain in athletes. Lower limb training is supposed to be more effective in progressing key rehabilitation outcomes, including knee extension strength, self-rated running capability, and running step length, when compared with lumbar stabilization exercises or back extensors exercises.

20.4.5 Medial Tibial Stress Syndrome

Approaching the MTSS rehabilitation treatment plan, an athlete and physical therapist should focus on static stretching of muscles involved into this overuse injury of lower leg—hamstring, gastrocnemius, and soleus.

20.4.6 Hamstring

For hamstring injury rehabilitation neuromuscular control as well as eccentric strengthening (PRES) and trunk stabilizing (PATS) exercises have been recommended. The primary aim of the rehabilitation program is reduction of pain and edema, restoration of proper neuromuscular control of lumbopelvic region at slower speeds and also prevention of excessive scar tissue formation while protecting the healing fibers from excessive lengthening. Achieving these goals, a patient is allowed to increase the intensity of exercise, neuromuscular training at faster speeds and larger amplitudes, and the initiation of eccentric resistance training. During the last phase advanced eccentric resistance training as well as high-speed neuromuscular training are implemented.

The main criteria for return to play in XC skiing are: (1) full, pain-free range of motion, (2) 80–90% of preinjury strength and endurance, (3) ability to maintain a neutral spine position while performing sport-specific exercises, plyometric exercises and sport-specific maneuvers without significant abnormal movement, (4) landing and cutting without compensation due to the injury.

20.5 Prevention Strategies

The key point to an injury prevention strategy in cross-country skiing is understanding the reasons that could lead to the injury. The factors hypothesized to contribute to the development of sports-related injuries can be divided into two categories: extrinsic and intrinsic factors.

All of those reasons could be divided into several categories: awareness, athlete's equipment, terrain, and general athlete training [3]. Previous injuries have also been shown to increase the risk of injury [5].

One of the most important parts of a prevention strategy is awareness of possible injuries, risk factors, and ways to avoid them. To provide better ankle stability, the use of high and hard boots is preferable. However, excessive support for the ankle joint could lead to an increase in boot-top fractures.

A prospective cohort study by Boyle et al. found that 88.4% of injuries occurred while skiing downhill. It is important to know and be able to control the speed while skiing downhill, and the ability to rotate a telemark was proposed as one of the solutions.

Focusing on technique and movement quality in the developing athlete could have a large impact on reducing injuries in the future (especially in cross training activities such as running and roller skiing).

A significant ($p = 0.011$) difference in the seasonal substantial injury prevalence was found for athletes that changed their ranking position between seasons [4].

Identifying existing problems (such as side differences in strength and balance) and assessing the junior athlete's movement competence to ensure it is appropriate for their sport may be important in preventing the first sport- or training-related injury [5].

References

1. Andersson E, Supej M, Sandbakk Ø, Sperlich B, Stöggl T, Holmberg H-C. Analysis of sprint cross-country skiing using a differential global navigation satellite system. Eur J Appl Physiol. 2010;110:585–95.
2. Sandbakk Ø, Holmberg H-C. A reappraisal of success factors for Olympic cross-country skiing. Int J Sports Physiol Perform. 2014;9:117–21.
3. Ristolainen L. Sports injuries in Finnish elite cross-country skiers, swimmers, long-distance runners and soccer players. Tiet Tutk ORTONin Julk A. 2011
4. von Rosen P, Floström F, Frohm A, Heijne A. Injury patterns in adolescent elite endurance athletes participating in running, orienteering, and cross-country skiing. Int J Sports Phys Ther. 2017;12:822.
5. Worth SG, Reid DA, Howard AB, Henry SM. Injury incidence in competitive cross-country skiers: a prospective cohort study. Int J Sports Phys Ther. 2019;14:237.

Tennis

21

Rosa López-Vidriero Tejedor, Michael Najfeld, and Emilio López-Vidriero

21.1 Characteristics of the Sport

Tennis was created in the nineteenth century by Harry Gem, and his friend Augurio Perera, who developed a game that combined elements of racquets and the Spanish-Basque ball game "pelota."

Nowadays, it is an Olympic sport played by millions of recreational players and is also a popular worldwide spectator sport.

It is a racket sport that can be played individually against a single opponent (singles) or between two teams of two players each (doubles).

It has the peculiarity that it can be played on a variety of surfaces. Grass, clay, and hard courts of concrete or asphalt topped with acrylic are the most common. Occasionally carpet is used for indoor play, with hardwood flooring having been historically used. Artificial turf courts can also be found.

Another characteristic is that tennis matches are not limited in duration by a predetermined length of play. Therefore, matches can often last several hours.

A match consists of a sequence of sets. The outcome is determined through a best of three or five sets system. On the professional circuit, men play best-of-five-set matches at all four Grand Slam tournaments, Davis Cup, and the final of the Olympic Games and best-of-three-set matches at all other tournaments, while women play best-of-three-set matches at all tournaments.

The four Grand Slam tournaments are: the Australian Open played on hard courts, the French Open played on red clay courts, Wimbledon played on grass courts, and the US Open also played on hard courts.

21.2 Physiological and Biomechanical Demands on Athletes

Success in tennis depends not only on the player's talent but also on the technique and biomechanics, which play an important role in stroke production.

The serving motion is a complex movement involving the whole body, and is developed and regulated through a sequentially coordinated and

R. López-Vidriero Tejedor (✉)
Sports Traumatology and Orthopaedic Surgery, ISMEC (International Sports Medicine Clinic), Seville, Spain

Arthroscopy Unit, Hospital Universitario Infanta Elena, Madrid, Spain

M. Najfeld
OCM München, Munich, Germany

E. López-Vidriero
Sports Traumatology and Orthopaedic Surgery, ISMEC (International Sports Medicine Clinic), Seville, Spain

G. L. Canata, H. Jones (eds.), *Epidemiology of Injuries in Sports*,
https://doi.org/10.1007/978-3-662-64532-1_21

task-specific kinetic chain of force development. An effective kinetic chain is characterized by three components: optimized anatomy, optimized physiology (flexibility, strength, and muscle activation), and optimized mechanics (sequential distributed forces).

The kinetic chain has some key points that are correlated with optimal force development and minimal applied loads; these include eight positions: foot placement (in line or foot back), knee flexion greater than 15°, counter-rotation with posterior hip tilt, controlled lordosis with an x-angle of 30° approximately, scapular retraction, good scapulohumeral rhythm with humeral horizontal abduction and humeral external rotation, back shoulder moving up and through the ball impact, then down into the follow-through, and finally, shoulder internal rotation and forearm pronation [1].

The most common points of pathomechanics include the legs, core, scapula, and shoulder. The kinetic chain works as a close system, and alteration in one segment creates changes within the entire system, triggering a cascade leading to injury. This is called the catch-up phenomenon, where changes in the interactive points modify/increase the forces in the distal segments, which often result in pain or injury.

21.3 Epidemiology of Injuries

Unlike other sports, tennis matches do not have a time limit and may vary from minutes to several hours. Tennis requires high aerobic and anaerobic demands, involving the whole kinetic chain (lower limbs, trunk and upper limbs) resulting in a range of injuries that can be chronic (caused by overuse) and acute traumatic injuries.

The most common tennis-related injuries are caused by overuse (61.4%) and mostly affect the upper limbs (45.9%), including rotator cuff tendinopathy, internal impingement, long head of the biceps tendinopathy, medial or lateral epicondylitis, tendininopathy and subluxation of the extensor carpi ulnaris tendon at the wrist, abdominal muscle strains, and disc degenerative pathologies [2].

Acute injuries affect mainly the lower extremities, such as ankle sprains, patellar or quadriceps tendinopathy, meniscal tears or hip injuries [2].

Epidemiological studies have been traditionally limited because there was no agreement for injury reporting. It was not until 2009 when a consensus statement was published to standardize documentation and study of tennis injuries [3]. This consensus recommends the use of 1000 match hours as the reporting frequency. The first study using this consensus by Sell et al. reported the injury trends form the US Open Tennis Championships from 1994–2009 and showed an overall rate of 48.1 injuries per 1000 match exposures (ME), with two ME per singles match and four for doubles match, with a higher rate of acute injuries (27.7 per ME) than chronic injuries (19.5 per ME), and most of them occurred during matches. The most common location for acute injuries was the ankle, followed by wrist, knee, foot, and shoulder. Among chronic overuse injuries, there were no big differences between the distribution of lower extremities (9.3 per ME) and upper extremities (8.2 per ME).

Overall, the most frequent location was the lower extremities (23 per ME), followed by upper extremities (17.7 per ME) and trunk (6.1 per ME).

McCurdie et al. reported the injury trends from Wimbledon, from 2003–2012, finding a total rate of 20.7 per 1000 sets played. 39% of injuries were acute, 34% acute-prior, 16% chronic and prior to the tournament and 11% recurrent injuries. They found a lower injury rate among male players compared to female players (17.7 vs. 23.4 per 1000 sets played).

Though the consensus recommended the use of 1000 match hours as the reporting incidence, these previous studies used data collected years before the statement, and match durations were not available from previous matches, consequently each study has used a different injury frequency, making direct comparisons difficult.

Focusing on chronic injuries, one of the most affected regions is the shoulder. Our study group has observed and studied that tennis players present changes on their shoulders due to overload and repetitive movements. Whether these changes are adaptive or pathological is not clear yet. This study group assessed a group of ATP/WTA **active** tennis players to evaluate the prevalence of injuries and these changes [4]. The study showed that 21.5% had shoulder injury in the last 3 months (14.1% of men and 40% of women). The vast majority of players (87.4%) had glenohumeral internal rotation deficit (GIRD), dyskinesis (57.7%), long head of the biceps (LHB) tenderness (35.5%), and tenosynovitis on the LHB by ultrasound (20%) on the dominant shoulder (Fig. 21.1a–d). Curiously, the mean external rotation (ER) was normal in both shoulders (93.8° on dominant and 93.3° on nondominant). Even if it seems that the nondominant shoulder might not suffer from these injuries/adaptive changes, it does; 56.3% had GIRD, 45.9% dyskinesis, 16.3% LHB tenderness, and 11.6% tenosynovitis on LHB on their contralateral shoulder. After the regression study, the predictive model of shoulder injury in the past 3 months showed that women had 4.3 ($p = 0.003$) times higher possibility of suffering an injury in the past 3 months ($p = 0.003$); those who have GIRD had 4.4 ($p = 0.008$) times lower possibility of injuries in the past 3 months than those without GIRD ($p = 0.008$). Participants with LHB tenderness presented 2.6 ($p = 0.05$) times higher possibility of injury than those without LHB tenderness, even if it was not statistically significant ($p = 0.051$). These results differ from those found on pitchers, where GIRD was found to be associated with increased shoulder pathology. It should be taken into account that tennis players have a normal ER, unlike pitchers, who have an increased ER. After these findings, it remains unclear whether GIRD is an adaptive change or a pathological one, but ER definitely plays an important role.

In a sub-study on the same population of active tennis players, suprascapular nerve entrapment was also observed, finding a prevalence of 7.5% in this cohort using a portable electroneurogram machine. In all of the cases, it appeared with atrophy of both the supraspinatus and infraspinatus fossae of the dominant shoulder (Fig. 21.1e, f), and it was correlated to higher age and amount of hours played of tennis. We theorize that it is related to a dynamic entrapment of the nerve due to the altered biomechanics of the scapula and shoulder complex found in our study.

Injuries to the elbow region involve mainly lateral and medial epicondylitis. Lateral epicondylitis or "tennis elbow" rate in recreational players is quite high, mainly because of the overload on the backhand ground stroke, ranging from 37–57%, while the incidence of medial epicondylitis is higher in elite players from overload on the serve and forehand strokes.

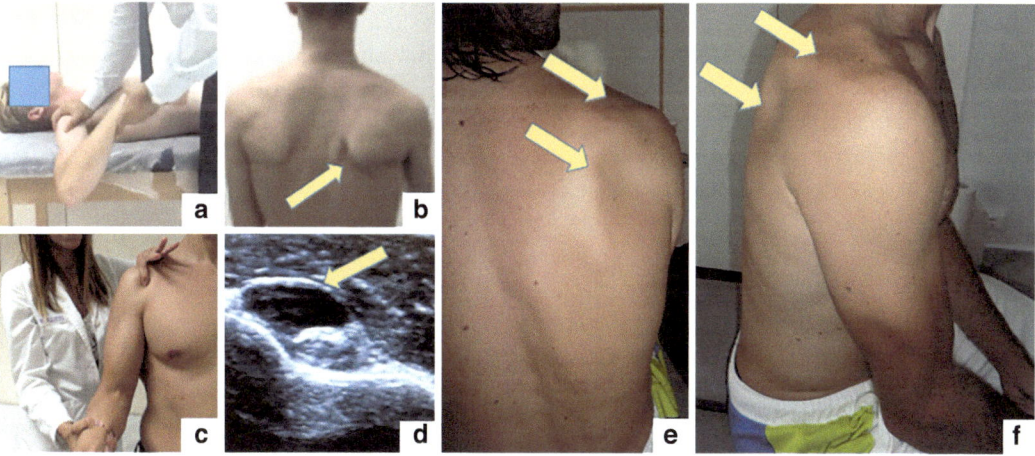

Fig 21.1 (**a**) GIRD, (**b**) Dyskinesis, (**c**) Long Head of the Biceps Tenderness, (**d**) Tenosynovitis on Long Head of the Biceps, (**e** and **f**) Supraspinatus and Infraspinatus atrophy secondary to Suprascapular Nerve entrapment

It is also important to highlight that tennis is played on different surfaces with different coefficient of friction and shock absorption which contributes to the injury rate and pattern of injury. Hard courts have the lowest shock absorption and highest coefficient of friction, leading to higher peak loads due to less sliding and shorter stopping distances. It should also be taken into account that ball speed is higher on these courts and may apply higher forces on the upper extremities. From Davis Cup data, 75% of the injuries happened on hard courts.

Contrariwise, clay courts have an increased shock absorption and lower coefficient of friction, decreasing the speed of the ball and are considered a slower surface. However, the lower coefficient of friction leads to more sliding, which might entail a different kind of injuries.

21.4 Specific Rehabilitation and Return to Play

The vast majority of the tennis players will respond to conservative treatment. The rehabilitation methods developed have become well researched and refined. One can use patient-directed assessment tools to categorize the injury in terms of the patient's sport and expectations. Measuring patient expectation, resiliency, and/or patient perceived function prior to the beginning of treatment can help provide insight to each individual patient's specific concerns and potential goals. Different tools exist to determine the player's specific goals, as well as pathways for rehabilitation and the right choice of it is guided by the patient's injury, as well as the athlete's needs.

Different approaches exist in the treatment of the most common upper extremity injuries of an athlete. The first step is to control the symptoms, which can be achieved with ceasing or decreasing the aggravating activity. The most common incapacitating pathology on the upper extremity in tennis players is pain from the long head of the biceps (LHB), which prevents them from serving, as well as creating difficulty with the volley and forehand. This first step consists of different

treatment protocols aiming at or around the site of injury with local application of corticoid mixed with local anesthetics. Other therapies can consist of radial shock, wave, platelet rich plasma (PRP) injections or percutaneous intratissue electrolysis with galvanic currents, all combined with physiotherapy [5]. All have in common the aim to ease the acute pain and bring relief to the athlete.

The second step consists of analyzing and treating the often underlying kinetic chain alterations. Several authors have described the concept of kinetic chain rehabilitation, and specifically in tennis this concept applies especially to chronic but also acute injuries. The comprehensive approach to the athlete's problem allows a more effective treatment plan, but also helps prevent the reoccurrence of the issue. This has been proven effective with specific injuries, scapula dyskinesis, as well as GIRD or posterior muscle tightness. Shoulder protocols have been designed according to studies and experience for whole muscle groups around the shoulder, with stretching areas, which are known to be tight for tennis players. Strengthening while controlling the muscles groups is another key element in a successful rehabilitation.

Scapular stability, dynamic stability of the glenohumeral joint, proprioceptive work, and the techniques of reintroducing the specific movements are all important. Mobility must be maintained as much as possible. It is therefore important to emphasize to the player the need to treat the underlying condition. Taking time to explain every exercise and correct the position and involving the tennis player team is mandatory to achieve good results. Furthermore, core strength and stability, energy transfer links for extremities, and closed chain exercises are key elements of a successful rehabilitation.

In terms of injuries, women suffer from more injuries than men, and it can be related to the number of matches they play (some months WTA tournaments/matches are twice the number of ATP tournament/matches). It can also be related to the higher frequency of hyperlaxity and instability in women.

Regarding the types of injuries related to the age of the tennis players, veteran players suffer more often from rotator cuff tears than younger players, especially in men (complete tears:18.8% vs 6.6%). In contrast to what is commonly seen in rotator cuff tears, fatty infiltration is rarely observed in tennis players.

Teenagers play with a lower level of physical conditioning, but fortunately, injuries in these players are usually not longstanding and the overuse (chronic) problems seen in older players, such as elbow epicondylitis or patellar/Achilles tendinopathy, are less common in young players. Anatomically, lower extremity injuries are twice as prevalent as those to the upper extremity or spine, with ankle sprain being the most common.

A comprehensive rehabilitation program takes into account the individual requirements of a tennis athlete as well as individual external, biological, and physiological factors that can influence a player's rehabilitation.

21.5 Prevention Strategies

There is the perception that higher training loads inevitably result in higher injury rates in athletes. Although it is true that high absolute training loads are associated with greater injury risk, there is also evidence that training may have a protective effect and that under training increases injury risk.

Multiple studies have identified alterations or changes in strength balance and muscle group performance in elite tennis players, which end up causing alterations in the kinetic chain, and therefore injuries. Thus, commonly injured areas should be targeted for preventive training strategies.

The prevention strategies are focused on resistive exercises for core, shoulder, elbow, hip, and lower extremity. To help develop successful prevention strategies, risk factors that prevent the return to play have to be identified. Changes to these individual factors are then often implemented together with the coach into the daily routine and exercises to avoid further harm to the player. Because tennis consists of a lot of repetitive movements, they need to be supervised vigorously by the coach or clinician assisting in the prevention.

As tennis is an asymmetric sport, the prevention strategies should also focus on achieving the most symmetric muscle-joint status as possible by working in the gym to strengthen and stretch the nondominant sides such as the contralateral upper extremity or the ipsilateral core muscles.

The movements required in tennis include repeated flexion, extension, lateral flexion, and rotation of the spine; therefore, extensive core stability training is critical to avoid back injuries and kinetic chain disorders. Warm up, flexibility, and strength are key elements in preventing injuries on any level of tennis.

For shoulder injuries prevention, rotator cuff and scapular and parascapular muscles exercises are essential. Most of the exercises explained in the rehabilitation program for shoulder injuries are also used in prevention programs.

Exercises recommended for prevention of elbow injuries are based on increasing the strength and muscle endurance of the wrist and forearm muscles.

Another important step in prevention injuries is regular movement analysis of the players to pick up weaknesses or unhealthy movement patterns, which could lead to an overuse injury. These steps should be realized together with the coach, who can implement changes to the technique, as well as training exercises to help prevent injuries and assure a good physical condition of the athlete.

Tennis remains an individual sport with specific demands to each player, and elite players rely mostly on their coaches, who shape their individual prevention programs. Different injury prevention programs for individual sports such as tennis have been developed, but none so far has been tested in a randomized controlled trial for its effectiveness. Success of a player nowadays is still measured by their ability to perform on a high level without major injuries.

References

1. Kibler WB, Wilkes T, Sciascia A. Mechanics and pathomechanics in the overhead athlete. Clin Sports Med. 2013;32(4):637–51.
2. Fu MC, Ellenbecker TD, Renstrom PA, Windler GS, Dines DM. Epidemiology of injuries in tennis players. Curr Rev Musculoskelet Med. 2018;11(1):1–5.
3. Pluim BM, Fuller CW, Batt ME, Chase L, Hainline B, Miller S, Montalvan B, Renström P, Stroia KA, Weber K, Wood TO, Tennis Consensus Group. Consensus statement on epidemiological studies of medical conditions in tennis, April 2009. Clin J Sport Med. 2009;19(6):445–50.
4. Lopez-Vidriero E, Lopez-Vidriero R, Gallardo E. The shoulder of professional tennis players: gird, tenosynovitis of biceps and dyskinesia. Knee Surg Sport Traumatol Arthrosc. 2014;22:S396.
5. Poberaj B, Taverna E, Dierickx C, Randelli P, Fossati C, López-Vidriero E, et al. In: Becker R, Kerkhoffs GMMJE, Gelber P, Denti M, Seil R, editors. Biceps tendinopathy (ICL2) ESSKA instructional course lecture book. Barcelona: Springer; 2016. p. 11–25.

Volleyball

22

Simone Cerciello, Katia Corona, Charles Fiquet, and Philippe Neyret

22.1 History of Volleyball

Volleyball, which is played by approximately 200 million players worldwide [1], was invented in 1895 by William G. Morgan, physical director of the Young Men's Christian Association (YMCA) in Holyoke, Massachusetts. It was intended as an indoor sport for those businessmen who found the game of basketball too vigorous. Morgan initially called it "mintonette," until a professor from Springfield College in Massachusetts noted the volleying nature of play and proposed the name of "volleyball." The original rules were written by Morgan and printed in the first edition of the Official Handbook of the Athletic League of the Young Men's Christian Associations of North America (1897). The game soon showed a wide appeal for both sexes in schools, playgrounds, the armed forces, and other organizations in the United States, and it was subsequently introduced to other countries.

In 1916, rules were issued jointly by the YMCA and the National Collegiate Athletic Association (NCAA). The first nationwide tournament in the United States took place in New York City in 1922. Volleyball was then introduced into Europe by American troops during World War I. At that time, the first national organizations were formed. The Fédération Internationale de Volley Ball (FIVB) was founded in Paris in 1947 and moved to Lausanne, Switzerland, in 1984. International volleyball competitions began in 1913 with the first Far East Games, in Manila. During the early 1900s and continuing until after World War II, volleyball in Asia was played on a larger court, with a lower net, and nine players on a team. The FIVB sponsored world volleyball championships for men in 1949 and for both men and women in 1952. Volleyball became an Olympic sport for both men and women at the 1964 Olympic Games in Tokyo.

22.2 The Game

The game is played on a 9 m (30 ft.) wide by 18 m (60 ft.) long court. A center line divides it into two equal playing areas for the two teams.

S. Cerciello (✉)
Casa di Cura Villa Betania, Rome, Italy

Marrelli Hospital, Crotone, Italy

K. Corona
Department of Medicine and Health Sciences "Vincenzo Tiberio", University of Molise, Campobasso, Italy

C. Fiquet
Clinique Protestante, Lyon, France

P. Neyret
Clinique Protestante, Lyon, France

Healthpoint, Abu Dhabi Knee & Sports Medicine Center, Abu Dhabi, United Arab Emirates

© The Author(s), under exclusive license to Springer-Verlag GmbH, DE, part of Springer Nature 2022
G. L. Canata, H. Jones (eds.), *Epidemiology of Injuries in Sports*,
https://doi.org/10.1007/978-3-662-64532-1_22

143

Players may not step completely beyond the center line while the ball is in play. A line is located 3 m (10 ft.) away and parallel to the center line on each half of the court and indicates the point in front of which a back court player may not drive the ball over the net from a position above the top of the net. This offensive action is called a spike and is usually performed most effectively and with greatest power near the net by the forward line of players. A tightly stretched net is placed across the court exactly above the middle of the center line; official net heights (measured from the top edge of the net to the playing surface—in the middle of the court) are 2.4 m (8 ft.) for men and 2.2 m (7.4 ft.) for women. A vertical tape marker is attached to the net directly above each side boundary line of the court, and, to help game officials judge whether served or volleyed balls are in or out of bounds, a flexible antenna extends 1 m (3 ft.) above the net along the outer edge of each vertical tape marker. The ball used is around 260–280 g (9–10 ounces) and is inflated to approximately 65 cm (25.6 in.) in circumference. A ball must pass over the net entirely between the antennae. A serve area, 9 m (30 ft.) long, is outside of each court end line. The serve must be made from within or behind this area. A space at least 2 m (6 ft.) wide around the entire court is needed to permit freedom of action, eliminate hazards from obstructions, and allow space for net support posts and the officials' stands. A clear area above the court at least 8 m (26 ft.) high is required to permit the ball to be served or received and played without interference. In competition, each team consists of six players, three of whom take the forward positions in a row close to and facing the net, the other three playing the back court. The 2000 Olympics introduced significant rule changes to international competition. One change created the *libero*, a player on each team who serves as a defensive specialist. The *libero* wears a different color from the rest of the team and is not allowed to serve or rotate to the front line. Another important rule change allowed the defensive side to score, whereas formerly only the serving team was awarded points.

22.3   Biomechanics of Volleyball

Volleyball is a high demanding sport with ankles, knees, and shoulders being the most solicited joints. The comprehension of the biomechanics of the specific skills allows better sport performance reducing the risk of injury. Jumping is the most important action of volleyball because it affects serving, spiking, and blocking and is closely related to landing. Jumping higher leads to increased performances [2]. Individual muscle properties, movement conditions, and jumping technique all influence the height of a jump.

The first aspect is muscle function; the force generated by the muscle is transferred trough the tendons to the bones and finally to the ground. These steps are influenced by muscle properties, composition of the tendons and the jumping surface (including both shoes and floor type). Intrinsic muscle properties such as the neural activation capacity, the force–velocity relationship, and the force–length relationship can be altered (within individual limits) by training. However training should be individualized to address and improve any specific neuromuscular system deficiencies: while some athletes might have to increase their maximal force development, others might have to improve upon a deficit in maximum muscle contraction velocity or maximum power capacity. Recent studies have confirmed that explosive plyometric training increases jump height in volleyball players [3].

The second aspect is the jumping technique; several aspects such as a countermovement or the arm swing may have substantial effects on jump height performance. A counter movement, i.e., a lowering of the center of mass just before the beginning of the push-off phase, can potentially increase jump height by approximately 7% [4]. The reasons for this increase are increased myoelectrical activity in the stretch–shortening cycle (SSC), the storage and recoil of elastic energy, and a higher active state, i.e., increased motoneuron activity before the start of the muscle shortening [5]. Researchers have also reported a 19–23% increase in jumping height due to the use of an arm swing. The reasons for this improvement are an elevated center of mass (due to arm elevation at take-off) and a decrease of contraction velocity of the leg muscle, which leads to an increase in muscle force generation via the force–velocity relationship.

The third aspect is the playing surface. It has been shown experimentally that jumps on sand are on average 14% lower than jumps from a rigid surface. The reason for this decrease is the energy absorbed by the sand. Similar but less substantial effects can be expected from different shoe soles or indoor surface materials. Although stiff materials have advantages during the take-off, they will also absorb less energy during the landing phase, which might lead to higher stress in the athlete's lower limb joints.

22.4 Epidemiology of Volley Injuries

The epidemiology of volleyball injuries is variable according to the level of athletes. The FIVB Injury Surveillance System analyzed 2640 of 2710 reports [6]. In total, 440 injuries were reported, 275 during match play (62.5%) and 165 during training (37.5%). The incidence of match injuries was 10.7/1000 player hours; this was greater for senior players than junior players (RR 1.32, 95% CI 1.03–1.69), while there was no difference between males and females (RR 1.09, 95% CI 0.86–1.38). The incidence of injuries during match play was greater for center players than for other player functions. The majority of injuries were minimal to mild, while severe injuries were rare; 10 of 440 injuries were expected to cause an absence of >4 weeks. Of these, eight occurred during match play, corresponding to an incidence of 0.3 severe injuries per 1000 player hours (95% CI 0.1–0.5). The ankle was the most commonly injured body part (25.9%), followed by the knee (15.2%), finger/thumb (10.7%), and lumbar/lower back (8.9%). This distribution was almost similar between match play (ankle 31.3%, knee 15.6%, fingers/thumb 10.2%) and training (ankle 17.0%, knee 13.2%, lower back 11.9%). The most common injury type was joint sprains (32.5%, $n = 143$), followed by muscle strains (14.1%, $n = 62$), and contusions (12.7%, $n = 56$).

Joint sprains affected mainly the ankle ($n = 87$), finger/thumb ($n = 26$), and knee ($n = 17$), while most muscle strains were located in the lower back ($n = 19$) and thigh ($n = 10$). In total, an ankle sprain was the most frequent specific diagnosis (19.8%). In total, 23.0% of all injuries ($n = 101$) were reported as the result of contact between players, while 20.7% ($n = 91$) were overuse injuries, and 17.3% ($n = 76$) were reported as noncontact trauma.

A Survey of Injuries Among Male Players of the Chinese Taipei National Volleyball Team showed that the incidence of injuries increased with the training sessions [7]. The percentage of incidences of injuries in the second session was greater than that in the first session when double sessions were performed daily. In the first session, 24%, 16%, 16%, and 16% of all injuries occurred in the knees, waists, fingers, and ankles, respectively. In the second session, knees and waists were the most common injury locations, which accounted for 33.3% and 23.8% of all injuries, respectively. Based on the statistics, knee injuries were the most severe and frequent injuries of the lower extremities, which accounted for 33.3% of all injuries, followed by waists (23.8%), ankles (16%), fingers (16%), and shoulders (12%).

A difference has been also recorded according to the different playing phase [8]. The authors reported a total of 178 injuries in 121 out of 144 volleyball players. The most common location was the ankle (23.03%) followed by knee (21.91%), shoulder (11.79%), back (10.67%), hamstring (9.55%), groin (6.74%), finger (6.17%), hand (3.93%), and other (5.61%).

The most common cause for injury was spiking (33.70%), blocking (24.15%), diving (17.41%), setting (11.23%), and other (14.04%). Maximum incidence of injuries affected muscles (32.40%), ligaments (24.71%), tendon (9.55%), bones (factures) (2.80%), braises (6.17%), and other (7.40%).

Among knee injuries, patellar tendinopathy, also known as "jumper's knee," is the most common situation having been reported in approximately 50% of male indoor volleyball players [9, 10]. The rate is slightly lower in elite players (approx. 40%) [11] and more frequent in males than females. It is more common in volleyball players who train on hard surfaces [11] and is therefore less common in beach volleyball players [12]. Middle blockers tend to suffer from jumper's knee more than do players at other positions.

On the contrary, acute trauma leading to anterior cruciate ligament (ACL) trauma is uncommon [13]. The reported incidence is approximately 0.1 ACL injuries/1000 athlete exposures among female collegiate volleyball athletes in the United States (compared with a rate of 0.4/1000 athlete exposures in soccer and 0.27/1000 athlete exposures in basketball) [14]. These data have been confirmed by retrospective cohort studies from Norway and the Netherlands [15, 16].

22.4.1 Prevention of Knee Injuries

Patellar tendinopathy is an overuse injury; symptom onset usually occurs gradually after a threshold of cumulative tissue injury has been exceeded. Histological examination on tendon samples reveals degeneration and fibrotic scarring of the tendon, particularly at the bone-tendon junction. The normally parallel collagen bundles are disorganized, and the observed tenocytes display altered morphology [17]. It has been hypothesized that excessive tendon loading induces tenocyte apoptosis (programmed cell death) [18]. An increased incidence of jumper's knee has been reported in athletes who jump highest and in those who develop the deepest knee flexion angle during landing from a spike jump [19]. Another study suggested that valgus knee strain during the eccentric loading phase of the spike jump take off may contribute to the observed asymmetric onset of patellar tendinopathy [10].

Potential prevention strategies include changes in the jumping technique, training, and rehabilitation.

Changes in the jumping technique in order to prevent valgus strain on the lead knee and to keep knee flexion to a minimum on landing may be advantageous in reducing the rate and severity of patellar tendinopathy. The importance of the landing phase of the jump must be highlighted because it is the most common reason for knee injuries in volleyball players. In any case, no clear scientific data have been published to support this fact.

Training volume on hard playing surfaces should not exceed the capacity of the patellar tendon to regenerate. However, it remains debated how often and by what percentage the volume of jump training can be safely increased over a given time period. It has been shown that a critical step occurs when young players are promoted from the junior to the senior level. During this passage, players are abruptly moved from a relatively safe training environment to an elite club or sports school that practices daily and has a structured program of weight training. Therefore, great care should be taken from muscle stretching and rest to strengthening. In addition, lack of strength and flexibility in the core muscles [20], and lack of balance or control of the body when jumping and landing, has been associated with poor form in the athlete's jumps resulting in injury and reduced performance.

Eccentric training protocols (particularly those using decline squats) have shown to be effective in treating patellar tendinopathy [21, 22]. However, other studies have reported that eccentric training of the quadriceps was ineffective in treating symptomatic jumper's knee in volleyball players during the competition season [23]. There is preliminary evidence that such knee extensor eccentric training protocols, used prophylactically, can effectively prevent sports related anterior knee pain from patellar tendinopathy [24]. Specific rehabilitation and strengthening of the core muscles may prevent functional imbalances of the lower limbs weakness contributing to the treatment of anterior knee pain. In addition, when treating jumper's knee, it is important to rehabilitate beyond the absence of symptoms, and to avoid return to play before the athlete is adequately rehabilitated, in order to maximize secondary prevention of recurrent injury and thus minimize the risk of chronicity.

Finally, although reports of benefit of external orthoses abound, there is no evidence to support the routine use of patellar straps (ostensibly designed to redistribute the forces acting on the patellar tendon) in the treatment or prevention of jumper's knee.

22.5 Conclusions

Volleyball is a common sport worldwide. Although it is a non contact sport, players often sustain knee injuries. They may result from direct trauma or overuse. Direct trauma may affect ACL, thus leading to instability, which inevitably requires surgical treatment. Overuse syndromes such as patellar tendinopathy are more common. They are caused by extrinsic (hard surfaces, shoes, training methods) or intrinsic (muscle performance, jumping technique, core muscle weakness) factors. Prevention is essential to reduce the severity of these injuries; however, when they occur, specific rehabilitation strategies and modifications of training programs are mandatory to achieve good results and return to performance.

References

1. Fédération Internationale de Volleyball (FIVB). Lausanne Switzerland: X-Press; 1994, 47:1.
2. Sattler T, Hadžić V, Derviševič EG, et al. Vertical jump performance of professional male and female volleyball players: effects of playing position and competition level. J Strength Conditioning Res. 2015;29(6):1486–93.
3. Ziv G, Lidor R. Vertical jump in female and male volleyball players: a review of observational and experimental studies. Scand J Med Sci Sports. 2010;20(4):556–67.
4. Wagner H, Tilp M, von Duvillard SP, et al. Kinematic analysis of volleyball spike jump. Int J Sports Med. 2009;30(10):760–5.
5. Bobbert MF, Gerritsen KG, Litjens MC, et al. Why is countermovement jump height greater than squat jump height? Med Sci Sports Exerc. 1996;28(11):1402–12.
6. Bere T, Kruczynski J, Veintimilla N, et al. Injury risk is low among world-class volleyball players: 4-year data from the FIVB Injury Surveillance System. Br J Sports Med. 2015;49(17):1132–7. https://doi.org/10.1136/bjsports-2015-094959.
7. Huang H-Y, Teng T-L, Liang C-C. Volleyball injuries: a survey of injuries among male players of the Chinese Taipei national volleyball team. Am J Sports Sci. 2015;3(6):109–14. https://doi.org/10.11648/j.ajss.20150306.12.
8. Jadhav KG, Deshmukh PN, Tuppekar RP, et al. A survey of injuries prevalence in varsity volleyball players. J Exerc Sci Physiother. 2010;6(2):102–5.
9. Reeser JC, Agel J, Dick R, et al. The effect of changing the centerline rule on the incidence of ankle injuries in women's collegiate volleyball. Int J Volleyball Res. 2001;4:12–6.
10. Lian OB, Engebretsen L, Bahr R. Prevalence of jumper's knee among elite athletes from different sports: a cross-sectional study. Am J Sports Med. 2005;33:561–7.
11. Ferretti A. Epidemiology of jumper's knee. Sports Med. 1986;3:289–95.
12. Bahr R, Reeser JC. Injuries among world-class professional beach volleyball players. The Federation Internationale de Volleyball beach volleyball injury study. Am J Sports Med. 2003;31:119–25.
13. Ferretti A, Papandrea P, Conteduca F, et al. Knee ligament injuries in volleyball players. Am J Sports Med. 1992;20:203–7.
14. NCAA. Injury Surveillance System. 2005. http://www1.ncaa.org/membership/ed_outreach/health-safety/iss/index.html. Accessed 19 Sep 2005.
15. Bahr R, Bahr IA. Incidence of acute volleyball injuries: a prospective cohort study of injury mechanisms and risk factors. Scand J Med Sci Sports. 1997;7:166–71.
16. Verhagen EA, Van der Beek AJ, Bouter LM, et al. A one season prospective cohort study of volleyball injuries. Br J Sports Med. 2004;38:477–81.
17. Cook JL, Feller JA, Bonar et al. (2004) Abnormal tenocyte morphology is more prevalent than collagen disruption in asymptomatic athletes' patellar tendons. J Orthop Res 22:334–338.
18. Scott A, Khan KM, Heer J, et al. High strain mechanical loading rapidly induces tendon apoptosis: an ex vivo rat tibialis anterior model. Br J Sports Med. 2005;39:e25.
19. Richards DP, Ajemian SV, Wiley JP, et al. Knee joint dynamics predict patellar tendinitis in elite volleyball players. Am J Sports Med. 1996;24:676–83.
20. Sommer HM. Patellar chondropathy and apicitis, and muscle imbalances of the lower extremities in competitive sports. Sports Med. 1988;5:386–94.
21. Young MA, Cook JL, Purdam CR, et al. (2005) Eccentric decline squat protocol offers superior results at 12 months compared with traditional eccentric protocol for patellar tendinopathy in volleyball players. Br J Sports Med. 2005;39:102–5.
22. Jonsson P, Alfredson H. Superior results with eccentric compared to concentric quadriceps training in patients with jumper's knee: a prospective randomised study. Br J Sports Med. 2005;39:847–50.
23. Visnes H, Hoksrud A, Cook J, Bahr R. No effect of eccentric training on jumper's knee in volleyball players during the competitive season: a randomized clinical trial. Clin J Sport Med. 2005;15:227–34.
24. Fredberg U, Bolvig L. Prophylactic training reduces the frequency of jumper's knee but not Achilles tendinopathy. Br J Sports Med. 2005;39:384.

Water Polo

23

Yigit Umur Cırdı and Mustafa Karahan

23.1 Characteristics of the Sport

Water polo originated in Britain and then became popular in Scotland. The rules of the game are influenced from football. The ball was originally called "pulu" which was made in India. This name evolved in time to "polo" and inspired the contemporary name of the sport. When water polo was accepted into the Olympic Games and gained international popularity, an official federation was initiated to manage official competitions, rules, and international connections between clubs.

The size of the field is 30 m × 20 m and depth of the pool must be at least 2 m. One team includes 13 players total, 7 players in field (1 goalkeeper +6 players) and 6 players as substitutes. Holding or carrying the ball with two hands is a foul and only the goalkeeper is allowed to handle the ball with two hands. Players are not allowed to touch the bottom of the pool. Duration of the game is 32 min total, and it is played in 4 quarters, with 8 min for each. Each team has 30 s on offense; if the shot clock is violated, possession passes to the other team.

Water polo demands enormous level of activity requiring endurance, stamina, and timely bursts of power. Players should be able to combine swimming, shooting, tackling, and frequent bursts of swimming sprints during competition. There is a continuous loop of frequent burst of approximately 15 s followed by reduced intensity episodes less than 20 s. Which makes water polo a highly stamina demanding collision sport with frequent physical contact. In addition to the physical contact, players must perform other crucial activities such as defending, shooting, blocking, jumping, and elevation from the water. All these activities together require high-profile body strength, agility, and robust body structure with tactical and technical capability.

23.2 Physiological and Biomechanical Demands on Athletes

Water polo demands neuromuscular strength and quickness during swimming to perform specific moves. Shooting is a crucial skill in water polo and essential for victory. The ball must be thrown with highest possible velocity and accuracy to score. Throwing in water polo is a modified overhead activity; therefore, few additional body movements are required. Because the area lacks solid ground to provide support for throwing,

Y. U. Cırdı
Department of Orthopedic Surgery, Acıbadem
Kozyatağı Hospital, Istanbul, Turkey

M. Karahan (✉)
Department of Orthopedic Surgery, Acıbadem
Mehmet Ali Aydınlar University School of Medicine,
Istanbul, Turkey

© The Author(s), under exclusive license to Springer-Verlag GmbH, DE, part of Springer Nature 2022   149
G. L. Canata, H. Jones (eds.), *Epidemiology of Injuries in Sports*,
https://doi.org/10.1007/978-3-662-64532-1_23

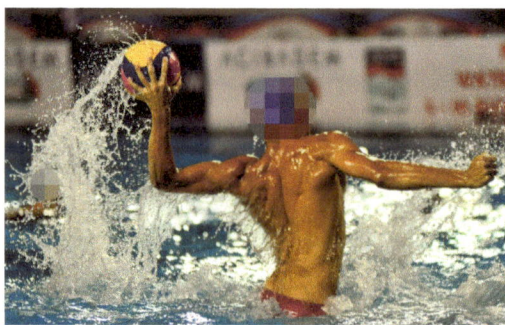

Fig. 23.1 Note the positioning of the ball and prominent rotation of the trunk

force is generated by a compensatory mechanism to reach max efficiency. The ball is positioned at the back of the head and trunk to generate most efficient power arch in the initiation phase. During the throwing phase, the arm is abducted from the trunk to produce greater angular momentum (Fig. 23.1). Trunk rotation is the major source of power to be delivered in the chain of motion (phases of throwing: preparation, cocking, acceleration, follow-through). For this reason, the trunk must be elevated vertically from the level of water to supply the player free shoulder movement and maximum lateral rotation (angular momentum). The vertical kick provides this elevation to raise the body out of the water and is known as an "eggbeater" kick. The speed of a shot in water polo may reach up to 80 km/h.

Swimming is a fundamental skill required in water polo. Significant endurance is required inside the water to perform key defensive and offensive duties during the competition. Players require excellent endurance, power, speed and condition. These specifications are not only essential during the competition but also required to complete long tournaments successfully. The defenders game style is relatively static, and they wrestle much more when compared with the offenders. Sprinting, endurance and agility is the key specifications for offenders and are directly related to offensive impact. Depending on the different demands of the individual, a specific training program should be prepared to provide athletes adequate physical strength to overcome this highly intense competition.

23.3 Epidemiology of Injury

23.3.1 Injury Patterns

Eight teams of National Water Polo League of Turkey have been studied. Two out of the eight teams refused to share sport specific injury data. Thus, 99 players of six different teams were followed for injuries throughout the season and post-season play-offs. A total of 170 matches were played in season (112) and play-offs (58). Therefore, 2380 player matches were played in the regular season, which corresponds to 1269.3 match hours. Fourteen injuries have been reported; 85.7% of injuries occurred due to contact with another player and 14.2% were secondary to overuse. Interestingly, the majority of injuries (71.4%) occurred during training, and 73.3% of these injuries were secondary to body contact. Most of the injuries did not result in game loss, except one broken rib, which resulted in absence for two consecutive matches during the competition, and 14.2% were during training; 80% of all injuries occurred due to contact with another player.

23.3.2 Injury Locations

Multiple body parts are involved in water polo, and they must work in harmony to perform complex tasks in water such as overhead movements, defending, eggbeater kicking, and swimming sprints. The demand of constant endurance and tense physical contact predisposes to a wide range of injuries from overuse injuries to acute high-energy traumas (Fig. 23.2). The most frequently encountered injuries are briefly summarized below.

23.3.2.1 Head
The head almost always stays above the water level both during the resting state and wrestling in the competition. Therefore, it is the most exposed body part and prone to injury. According to the regulations by FINA (Federation Internationale de Natation), players can wear only a swimming cap with protective ear covers to block direct trauma to the ear and ear drum. In case of the per-

Head

- Contusion
- Concussion
- Dental inuries
- External otitis (swimmers ear)
- Rupture of the ear drum
- Blow-out fracture
- Corneal abrasion

Upper Extremity

- Rotator Cuff Tear
- Biceps Tendinitis
- Labral injuries (Bankart lesion, SLAP lesion)
- Ulnar Collateral ligament sprain/rupture
- Osteochondritis Dissecans (OCD)
- deQuervain's tenosynovitis
- Phalangeal, metacarpal fractures and dislocations
- Lacerations
- Web space tear
- Gamekeeper's thumb
- Shoulder instability
- Scapular dyskinesis

Lower Extremity

- Groin pain
- Pubalgia
- Hamstirng strain
- Meniscus tear
- Femoroacetabular impidgement
- Collateral ligament strain
- Trochanteric bursitis
- Iliotibial band syndrome
- Ankle impidgement
- Muscle Cramps

Trunk and Miscellaneous

- Cervical ligament
- Sternal fracture
- Degenerative disc disease
- Radiculopathy
- Chronic rhinitis
- Wheezing
- Cough
- Dermatologic lesions
- Tinea pedis (athlete's foot)
- Molloscum contagiosum (water warts)
- Skin irritation
- Melanoma

Fig. 23.2 List of common injuries in water polo

foration of the drum, player should be kept away from the water until recovery. The main purpose of the cap is to enable players to discriminate team members and opponents. The cap works more like a team identifier, and it has very limited protection ability for head trauma. This lack of actual protection makes the head and face prone to injuries such as laceration, fractures, and contusions. The head is the most affected part of the body according to recent large observational studies (25.6% of all injuries) [1]. Head injuries range from simple lacerations to contusions depending on the severity of the impact. Concussion is a severe injury that may progress to a life-threatening situation if unrecognized; 36% of players suffer from concussion at least one time during their career depending on the position of the player and gender. It is also shown that goalies are at higher risk for concussion.

Dental injuries are investigated as a subgroup of head injuries. It is reported that 21% of Swiss water polo players suffered at least one tooth injury during their career, which cannot be overlooked [2]. Usage of a mouth guard on a regular basis should be taken into consideration.

23.3.2.2 Upper Extremity

Lacerations are frequently observed due to contact with opponent and mostly seen in the hand. Fingernails of the opponents may cause skin cuts, abrasions, or lacerations during wrestling for the ball. Actual prevalence of this kind of injury is under-reported because most of them are neglected by the players.

Hand was the second most commonly injured body part in FINA World Championship and Olympic games (16.1%) and upper extremity was the most frequent site. Hands are prone to injury during the struggle for the ball. Many different injury mechanisms may result in the hand such as over-stretching, shooting, blocking the high velocity ball, and blunt trauma. Collateral ligament sprains, skin lacerations, dislocations, and even fractures might be observed. There might be correlation between the ball size and frequency of the injuries in hands because the water polo ball is relatively larger. Elbow and wrist injuries are relatively less common. Most elbow and wrist injuries are contusions and laceration. In addition, careful evaluation of the ulnar collateral ligament of the elbow is necessary, especially in shooters.

Shoulder injuries are quite common in water polo and investigated extensively. Reported incidence rates of shoulder injury range between 25 and 51% according to a recent systematic review [3]. Due to the intense repetitive action of overhead activity and continuous swimming, the shoulder joint is prone to injury in almost every moment of the game. Many distinctive actions in water polo put pressure on the shoulder joint such as swimming sprint, throwing a large ball, blocking, and wrestling with an opponent. The burden of the high demand activities on the shoulder joint is the reason for the frequent acute or chronic shoulder pain in athletes. Development of internal impingement and rotator cuff tears are associated with this feature. More severe injuries can also be observed such as subluxations and dislocations secondary to acute trauma. It has to be kept in mind that etiology of shoulder pain is multifactorial and should be followed closely.

23.3.2.3 Lower Extremity

Continuous swimming endurance and burst of sprints requires both aerobic and anaerobic training. Players must gain adequate stamina to complete both "head up" and "head down" swimming tasks. In water polo, strength of the lower extremity is closely associated with athletic performance. Vertical propelling force is generated by powerful kicking of the lower limb (eggbeater kick). This vertical elevation provides basic stance position above the water to perform essential tasks such as shooting, passing, grappling and blocking. Medial collateral ligament strains, hip and groin injuries, and meniscal tears may occur while performing these moves. Training with weight attached jackets and weight carrying drills are the most preferred techniques to strengthen quadriceps and hamstring muscle groups.

23.4 Treatment, Rehabilitation and Return to Play

Water polo is a tough sport and demands fitness and strength all across the board. Several injuries are observed depending on the body part involved. Therefore, an individualized treatment plan and rehabilitation program should be prepared depending on the index injury, which requires different specialists to be involved in the healing phase. The aim of the treatment and rehabilitation is restoring the athlete's activity level to the same level prior to injury and minimizing the number of games missed. A customized rehabilitation program is followed to fulfill athletic needs. Cooperation between the physician and physiotherapist is essential to prepare the athlete for competition. The physician must be aware of every step in players athletic recovery stage to adjust intensity of the training if needed.

Unfortunately, severe injury to the head may result in undesirable conditions such as concussion. Thus, signs of the concussion must be recognized immediately by the team physician, coach, and other players to prevent the advancing of the symptoms. In this case, the player should be taken out of the pool immediately and undergo an evaluation by a healthcare professional.

Shoulder injuries are the most common sports-related injury in water polo. Muscles included in the process of throwing should be improved and strengthened proportionally. Otherwise, an imbalance between upper extremity muscle groups leads to transformed throwing biomechanics and reduces the durability threshold against injury [4]. The etiology of the shoulder injury is often multifactorial; therefore, post-treatment protocol should be adjusted addressing the underlying pathology. A combination of exercises for strengthening and stretching are most beneficial.

Due to the tough nature of water polo, athletes are exposed to continuous grappling and body contact. Vigorous training and repetitive movements such as throwing, defending, and blocking cause fatigue on muscles and ligaments, making the occurrence of overuse traumas inevitable. Management of overuse traumas are relatively different than most of the acute injuries. Because the index injury is caused by chronic stress on the affected tendon and muscle, conservative treatment such as resting, ice compress, and immobilization is adequate. However, it is much more efficient to prevent overuse traumas prior to occurrence without causing game loss. Appropriate strengthening of the effected structure is necessary to avoid recurrence.

Most of the miscellaneous injuries in water polo are associated with increased duration of exposure to water. Infectious and non-infectious skin lesions are not uncommon. Warts and sores of the skin should not be underestimated and unusual skin lesions should be presented to the specialist. Chlorinated water is an irritant for eyes and associated with headache. Therefore, the quality of the water regarding pollution and the amount of chemicals should always be between the particular limits.

In conclusion, water polo is a rough sport, and it may be challenging to deal with the wide variety of injuries. High physiologic demand and regular close contact lead to increased frequency of overuse trauma. Close follow up and a suitable training program is essential to decrease the burden of injuries on the team.

23.5 Prevention Strategies

- Concussion is a serious injury in water polo and should be recognized immediately. Athletes experiencing severe head trauma must be taken out of the pool. Team members and staff should be trained for the possible scenario.
- Mandatory usage of mouth guards should be taken into consideration.
- Comprehensive injury surveillance is required to address underlying causes of overuse injuries other than trauma.
- Video surveillance would be beneficial to detect brutality and should be introduced to all athletes.
- Fair play is crucial for water polo. Emphasis should be given to these programs to prevent sport injuries.

References

1. Mountjoy M, Miller J, Junge A. Analysis of water polo injuries during 8904 player matches at FINA World Championships and Olympic games to make the sport safer. Br J Sports Med. 2019;53(1):25–31.
2. Hersberger S, et al. Dental injuries in water polo, a survey of players in Switzerland. Dent Traumatol. 2012;28(4):287–90.
3. Miller AH, et al. Shoulder injury in water polo: a systematic review of incidence and intrinsic risk factors. J Sci Med Sport. 2018;21(4):368–77.
4. Stromberg JD. Care of water polo players. Curr Sports Med Rep. 2017;16(5):363–9.

Wrestling

24

Szabolcs Molnár, Károly Mensch, Katalin Bacskai,
Éva Körösi, Ákos Sántha, and Krisztián Gáspár

24.1 Characteristics of the Sport

Wrestling is one of the most demanding sports of mind, spirit, and physical stamina [1, 2]. It is very complex. Athletes may meet anaerobic condition during a match, aerobic condition during a competition, and they need appropriate technical and tactical skills [3]. It is both a contact and collision sport, putting extreme demands on the entire body, which often results in injury [4]. In addition, inadequate preparation or the smallest lapse in concentration can also facilitate injury [5, 6].

The governing body of Olympic wrestling is the United World Wrestling (UWW) [7]. The Health Regulations of the UWW are very clear and are under continuous supervision by the Medical Commission [8]. There are also well prepared medical instructors, doctors, and health care providers both for the UWW and for the National Federations, who are present at adult international competitions [9]. There is a well-established surveillance system with continuous education for referees, coaches, local medical teams, and venue doctors [10].

S. Molnár (✉)
Department of Traumatology, Medical Centre
Hungarian Defence Forces, Budapest, Hungary

University of Physical Education, Budapest, Hungary

Medical, Prevention & Anti-Doping Commission of
United World Wrestling, Corsier-sur-Vevey,
Switzerland
e-mail: molnar.szabolcs.lajos@hm.gov.hu

K. Mensch
Department of Oral Diagnostics, Faculty of Dentistry,
Semmelweis University, Budapest, Hungary
e-mail: mensch.karoly_frigyes@dent.semmelweis-
univ.hu

K. Bacskai
National Institute for Sports Medicine, Budapest,
Hungary
e-mail: bacskai.katalin@osei.hu

É. Körösi
Hungarian Wrestling Federation, Budapest, Hungary
e-mail: korosie@birkozoszov.hu

Á. Sántha
Professional Medical Services and Assistance Ltd.,
Budapest, Hungary
e-mail: drsantha@halthguardhungary.com

K. Gáspár
Department of Dermatology, University of Debrecen,
Debrecen, Hungary
e-mail: gaspar.krisztian@med.unideb.hu

G. L. Canata, H. Jones (eds.), *Epidemiology of Injuries in Sports*,
https://doi.org/10.1007/978-3-662-64532-1_24

24.2 Physiological and Biomechanical Demands on Athletes

Wrestling is a very dynamic sport with several challenges and even well-prepared athletes may become prone to injuries. In spite of being traditional and popular, because of its complexity, sometimes the injury mechanism and pattern are hardly comprehensible of those medical personnel who are not familiar with them [6].

The highly demanding physical preparation of a wrestler is complicated by the different dietary regimens that must be followed during the training period, for weight loss or competition. Rapid weight loss enhanced by other risk factors can contribute to injuries [11–13].

Though the bouts and training sessions take part on soft mats along with an increasing number of precautions and improvements to defend wrestlers, injuries remain inevitable [14]. One independent key is the biomechanical aspect of wrestling mats, which also plays a major role in minimizing the rate and severity of injuries [6].

24.3 Epidemiology of Injuries

Comparing the incidence of injury among studies is difficult because of the variable ways "injury" has been defined and due to the different rate calculation methods [15, 16].

In wrestling, the number of injuries is relatively higher than in other sports considering the number of competitors. One study about the epidemiology of injuries among young male wrestlers (aged 7–17 years) from 2000 to 2006 demonstrated that 75% of the injuries occurred in the upper body, 97% of them were minor, and thus the wrestlers were discharged from the hospital soon after the accidents [17]. The injury rate per calendar year among college wrestlers was reported between 4.4 and 10.1/1000 exposed hours in different school years [18]. Approximately 8% of all injuries required surgical treatment [19]. The injury rate during competitions among wrestlers aged 6–16 years was 12.7%, and in 4.6% of those,

the wrestler had to give up the competition earlier than expected [20].

24.3.1 The Types of Wrestling Injuries

These include concussions, bleedings, abrasions, wounds, strangulation, contusions, muscles strains, joint sprains, dislocations, fractures, spinal shock, and paresis. Concussions and other head injuries account for 1–8% of all wrestling injuries [15]. Bleedings, abrasions and wounds are common injuries representing the major part of all injuries; skin lacerations approximately 40%, nose bleedings 18%, and skin contusions 10% [10]. Biting injuries may need special surgical consideration with occasional tetanus vaccination.

24.3.2 Timing and Onset

These are also important factors, and the following characteristics must be carefully considered. It should be noted, when exactly the injury occurred:

- In preseason or during the season;
- In which part of the bout or training: first or second period of bouts, early or late part of training;
- Whether it is an acute or chronic problem, overuse or re-injury.

24.3.3 Severity

- Mild, which is treated fully on the mat,
- Moderate, which is treated primarily on the mat but needs more attention and the athlete is referred to medical personnel at the venue.
- An injury is considered severe if it resulted in termination of the bout and/or needs hospital transfer [10].
- Critical (catastrophic), which may pose a threat to life or may lead to grave permanent disability. Most of them involve severe rota-

tional or axial blows to the cranial and cervical region that can result in fractures or dislocations with or without head trauma [15].

- The rate of direct catastrophic injury in the USA was reported between 0.72 and 0.97 per 100,000 wrestlers in college or high school competitions [21]. Forty-two percent of the injuries occurred during takedown and 71% during matches [22]. Another study revealed that 50% of the 24 catastrophic injuries involved the cervical spine, spinal cord or head [23]. In addition to full recovery, there were permanent disability, transient quadriplegia, severe head injuries, herniated disc, and death among the consequences [22].

24.3.4 Body Regions and Parts

The different studies rate the injuries' location by body region: head/spine/trunk (range of 24.5–48%), upper extremity (range of 9.3–42%), lower extremity (range of 7.5–45.1%), and the skin (range of 5–21.6%) [15].

24.3.4.1   Head and Neck

- **Neck soft tissues.** Strangulation injury—with illegal headlock one could suffer loss of consciousness, due to compression to the trachea, carotid artery, or carotid bulb causing bradycardia via vagus reflex. It may seem horrible but with proper first aid actions recovery is fast. In case of any doubt, suspension from the competition and further hospital investigation may be required [24].
- **Cervical spine injury.** To avoid the most dangerous consequences of it, one has to follow the protocol of the so-called ABC rules. In former epidemiological studies, neck injuries make up 0.8–14.9% of the total number [15].
- **Nose.** Injuries to the nasal region range from 0.7% to 5.7% of the total. Fractures are rare [15].
- **Cauliflower ears.** This is the special "trademark" of the wrestlers. Bleeding of the cartilage produces a blood clot under the perichondrium and results in the formation of fibrous tissue [9]. They may occur with the headgear on, but mostly when the head is

unprotected. In an early study, only 2 of 49 high school coaches (4.1%) required their wrestlers to wear headgear in the USA [25].

- **Eye.** The lesion of the cornea is very common but not serious. Characteristic symptoms are tearing and the inability to keep the eyes open (blepharospasm). It is advised to rinse and cover the injured eye as well as refer the wrestler to the closest ophthalmology department [26]. Ocular trauma rates are very low in the former epidemiological studies. Serious injuries are very rare, only two cases of blowout (elbow and knee to eye) are reported [15].
- **Orofacial region.** The most commonly affected are the front teeth, their periodontium, and the surrounding soft tissues (e.g., lips, tongue, cheeks). For severe dental trauma, oral surgery consultation is often necessary to make the wrestler able to continue the competition on the next day. A study at seven high schools during one school year found that 69.9% of wrestlers sustained some type of orofacial injury. Most of these were lacerations and contusions. Dental injuries in this study accounted for 10% of the total [27].

Upper extremity. Injuries have been reported anywhere from 9.3 to 42% of the total. The shoulder had the biggest proportion, as high as 24% of all reported injuries. The upper arm had the lowest reported frequency ranging from 0.8 to 1.4% [15]. The most frequent injury types included glenohumeral subluxation or dislocation, ulnar collateral ligament tears at the elbow, shoulder impingement, and acromioclavicular joint sprains, although there were significant variations. First year college wrestlers in the USA suffered a significantly higher percentage of shoulder and elbow injuries than more senior athletes, signifying an association between experience and risk of injury. There is a four-fold higher incidence of injury during competition. Injuries were significantly more likely to occur later in the match, with a 2.5-fold increased risk compared with early. While 26.8% of wrestlers were out of play for at least 14 days, only 5.9% of them required surgery [28].

- **Sternoclavicular joint.** Dislocation here is relatively frequent in wrestling but not very serious. Generally, 1 week of rest for recovery is sufficient [6].
- **Collar bone.** Children are more prone to fractures. Rarely needs surgical intervention [6].
- **Acromioclavicular joint.** Very often damaged, mostly Rockwood I or II dislocation. Rockwood III and IV are complete tears, and type IV surgery is always the treatment [6].
- **Shoulder girdle.** Bankart lesion requires surgical stabilization or Latarjet procedure. Posterior instability necessitates arthroscopic anchor screws. Shoulder injuries have been reported in the range of 3.5–24% of all, and it is second only after knee [15].
- **Biceps.** Very frequently injured. SLAP (superior labrum anterior and posterior) lesion or long head rupture. It needs reinsertion or tenodesis [29].
- **Pectoral muscle.** In general, it does not need intervention, ranges from 11.5% to 57% considering wrestler to all athletes ratio in different studies [30, 31].
- **Elbow.** Very common and typical site of injury in wrestling. The incidence of elbow injuries is higher than in other sports. Sometimes the diagnosis is difficult either due to late medical attendance or strong positioning muscles. Prolonged immobilization must be avoided to prevent development of a stiff elbow [32]. Dislocation, radial head fracture, collateral ligament injury and ulnar nerve dislocation are due to failed landing techniques or hyperextension during defensive maneuvers. One study revealed that elbow dislocation is unrelated to the wrestler's body weight, and 39% of the cases were associated with a previous injury [33].
- **Forearm, wrist and hand.** Frequent but usually minor injuries accounted for 1.2–11.2% of all. Gamekeeper's thumb or little joint sprain occur mostly and these damages are managed with taping [15].

Trunk: the incidence is 10% among wrestlers [34].

- **Chest, ribs and intercostal muscles.** Contusions are frequent, with temporary symptoms, and rapid recovery is expected. They comprise 4.1–16.1% of the total and can result from direct or indirect trauma. Most of them are contusions or costochondral sprains, but rib fractures are also common [15]. In case of sprain 3–6 weeks off is advised because this region may become painful for roll over in "par terre" position.
- **Abdomen.** Not typical. Abdominal injuries account for only 0.35–0.4% of the total number in wrestling [15].
- **Lumbar spine.** Low back pain is frequent both in active and retired wrestlers due to the load that it has to carry. They range from 1.2 to 18.6% of the total [15]. Spondylolysis and spondylolisthesis are typical, specifically of the L4 and L5 vertebrae in active wrestlers. Notably, 25–30% of the wrestlers presenting with lumbar pain had spondylolysis or spondylolisthesis, and 58% of them were diagnosed with lumbar strain [35]. Degenerative disc disease is common among retired wrestlers. The same symptoms can occur with different pathologies, which can cause difficulties achieving the correct diagnoses. Sometimes the sudden complaints originate from chronic degeneration [5].
- **Pelvis.** Atypical and infrequent, mostly occur to the pubic bones.

24.3.4.2 Lower Extremity
- **Muscles and tendons.** Partial rupture is frequent but does not require more than 2–4 weeks rest. Fortunately, it necessitates surgical intervention rarely, in certain cases of quadriceps muscle or Achilles tendon tear [6].
- **Knee.** The knee is the most commonly affected body part, ranging from 7.6 to 18.7% of all wrestling injuries [15]. They are the most common season-ending injuries, representing 44% of the total; 21% of knee injuries lead to more than one week of absence from competition [36]. Common types include medial and lateral collateral ligament sprains, medial and lateral meniscus tears, and prepatellar bursitis. The most frequent are sprains, which make up 30–65% of the total number of knee injuries. Meniscal injuries are also common, with a relatively high proportion of

lateral compared to medial meniscus tears. In different studies, lateral meniscus injuries represented from 7% to 46% of the total number of meniscal injuries [15]. Although knee injuries appear to be very common in wrestling, ACL tears are not, comprising between 0% and 9.1% of all knee injuries [37]. The ACL injury is usually the result of a landing maneuver at a competition, where the loaded extremity's open kinetic chain suddenly changes for the closed. Partial meniscectomy takes 3–4 weeks for recovery, but the ACL reconstruction takes much longer. Prepatellar bursitis represents 21% of all knee injuries. Of the bursitis cases, 50% were recurrent injuries. Eight cases of septic bursitis were reported [39].

- **Ankle and foot.** The prevalence of the distortions is high, but they seldom need surgery. In prospective studies, ankle injuries range from 3.2 to 9.7% of all wrestling injuries. The most common is the lateral ligament sprain, which usually occurs during takedowns [15].

24.4 Rehabilitation and Return to Play

The "return to play" requires the same amount of time as recommended for general athletes. Generally, our suggestion is to complete a regular rehabilitation program and then to implement the sport specific rehab exercises. We need well prepared physiotherapists, who understand wrestling with its challenges and are able to approach it with our sport protocols.

24.5 Prevention Strategies

Targeting injury prevention must include surveillance (data on occurrence of injury), risk factor identification, intervention evaluation, and implementation. The UWW and the National Federations had used a paper-based feed-back system until 2016. Since then, a cloud base data collection system of the competitions has been implemented, where all documented injuries must be registered. The main risk factor is itself

the nature of wrestling. It is a contact combat sport with collision and extreme demands on the entire body [5]. The exposure time to injuries is also important: practice, competition, and years spent with wrestling. Further risk factors are the training methods (aerobic and anaerobic, conditioning, technical preparation, strength), whether protective equipment is used (head gear, knee pads, mouth guards), and the quality of the facilities (training hall, mat properties, rest, and medical facilities). It is essential to have proper staff of trainers, physiotherapists, masseur, medical team with a doctor, and nutritionist available for support. Fundamental elements are nutrition, hydration, dehydration, fasting, and weight loss methods. It is also important to pay attention to fatigue as well as to take care of circadian rhythm, sleeping, and proper regeneration after crossing time zones. The trainers should separate younger age wrestlers with significant age, weight, or competency difference [15].

Prevention strategies should include functional training, continuous development of the UWW health regulations, medical examinations before weigh-in, and match rules with medical importance. It is also important to know how to avoid injuries on the wrestling mat during competitions; therefore, we should educate the referees, trainers, local medical teams, and venue doctors in UWW organized clinics and conferences [6]. One essential, but often underemphasized factor is the compliance of the athlete. The trainer and the team leader should not convince the injured wrestler to continue or return early.

Our top priority in the UWW Medical Commission is to draw more attention to penalizing dangerous situations (brutal actions, strangulation, head butting, punching, kicking, twisting of leg, arm, and finger), to prevent rapid weight loss (by applying 10 weights and weigh-in on the same morning), to reduce overload of competitors (2 day competition), and to improve referee–doctor communication by UWW Medical Coverage Guideline and educational programs [8]. As a result of these efforts, the rate of wrestling injuries in the Olympic Games had been diminished gradually: 24.2% in 2004, 9.3% in 2008, 12% in 2012, and 6.2% in 2016 [10].

From the medical point of view, we would like to detail the following strategies:

24.5.1 Functional Training

Primary prevention is of utmost importance, where functional training is the key element. Wrestling-specific movements must be practiced, not only the general exercises. Most of the injuries could be avoided by carefully monitoring the load on the wrestlers and with wrestling specific functional training. These exercises promote primary prevention as well as rehabilitation after injuries or surgeries.

24.5.2 Equipment and Protection Considerations

Athletes spend the biggest part of their preparation period in training halls, where they practice on the wrestling mat. The quality of wrestling mats plays a major role in minimizing the rate and severity of injuries. The mats' main function is to provide a safe environment for dynamic wrestling and protect wrestlers from injuries that are related to landing or loads created by throws. There are well-defined laboratory measurement protocols for the mats, which are included in the UWW rules and regulations. Wrestling mats must be replaced or reconditioned when they become worn [6].

The training hall must have padded walls, obstacles such as columns or bleachers, inadequate space, extreme heat or humidity are obviously detrimental as well. Cleaning of the mats is also part of the daily routine. Without daily disinfection, counts of microorganisms on the mat will increase as does the risk of transmission of dermatological infections from mat to wrestler.

According to the UWW Medical Rules, all protecting gear and tapings used in a competition must be under the control and supervision of the Medical Commission, especially the doctor nominated for the competition. The device should not contain metal. The orthosis and the tape must be documented and approved before weigh-in [8]. Special devices include ear protector, dental guard, and orthodontic brace. The latter are popular and can prevent teeth and the surrounding soft tissue injuries without any discomfort. Elbow, wrist, thumb, knee, and ankle supports are also frequently used.

24.5.3 Health Regulations and Pre-weigh-in Medical Examination

- **The Health Regulations of the UWW** are very clear and are under continuous supervision by the Medical Commission. There are also well prepared medical instructors, doctors, and health providers both for the UWW and for the National Federations present at adult international competitions. Annual detailed medical examination of the athlete is obligatory, but clearance is also advised 3 weeks before the competition [8].
- **Pre-weigh-in medical examination:** the medical examination before competition is a very important final screening [9]. It is a general, approximately 30–60-second-long examination to recognize obvious ailments, such as open wounds, skin infections (e.g., dermatomycosis, verruca, impetigo), fever, arrhythmia, fracture or dislocation, contagious diseases of skin, hair, and nails. The inspection is obligatory and independent from the issued and valid sport medical license [8].

24.5.4 Diet for Wrestlers

Due to concerns about weight control, wrestlers notoriously tend to skip meals or restrict their daily food intake, which may negatively influence their performance and enhance the risk of injury [11, 13, 38]. In order to maintain the high energy levels needed for their intense workouts, wrestlers need to consume a healthy, balanced diet daily, on a regular basis. The ideal diet should contain 50% of carbohydrates, 20% of protein, and 30% of fat [6]. Another important element is fiber intake. From the youngest age group, children must be educated about the importance of the right nutrition. The supportive management (trainers, sport leaders) must learn and accept the natural growth and development of children and should not force them into any weight category, under the age of 18. Losing only 2% of the body weight may even result in a significant reduction of performance; therefore, between the competition and the training weight, there should not be a bigger than 5% difference [12].

There are three kinds of diets for athletes that should be promulgated: preparation, weight cutting, and competition diets. They all must be designed and harmonized according to the special nutritious demands of the given period.

24.5.5 Match Rules with Medical Importance

The UWW has a detailed Medical Regulation with Responsibilities of the doctor assigned to the competition. A Practical Medical Guide for Wrestling Competitions is prepared in order to help those physicians or health care providers who are not familiar either with the wrestling rules or with common wrestling injuries [9]. The UWW defined the basic steps for examination by medical professionals before the weigh-in (see above), the relation with the Chief Referee/Technical Delegate, as well as the behavioral standards on the mat (e.g., communication with the referees, trainers, and wrestlers). The typical medical issues and injuries of wrestling are also listed. Moreover, the various reasons and ways to suspend a bout are also strictly regulated [8]. The Medical Commission also developed a sign language among referees and doctors to ease the communication [6].

In case of injury, the competitor should not leave the mat, and the doctor has to decide if the wrestler can continue or needs further medical assistance. During the competition, if such position or situation that can be dangerous to a wrestler's health is observed, then in order to prevent further injury, the doctor can stop the bout, even if such event was left unnoticed by the referee [8].

References

1. Guttmann A. The olympics: a history of the modern games. Champaign, IL: University of Illinois Press; 2002.
2. Poliakoff M. Wrestling, freestyle. In: Levinson D, Christensen K, editors. Encyclopedia of world sport: from ancient times to the present, vol. 3. Santa Barbara, CA: ABC-CLIO; 1996. p. 1191. ISBN 0-87436-819-7.
3. Mirzaei B, Curby DG, Barbas I, Lotfi N. Physical fitness measures of cadet wrestlers. Int J Wrestling Sci. 2011;1(1):63–6.
4. Halloran L. Wrestling injuries. Orthop Nurs. 2008;27(3):189–92; quiz 193-4. PMID: 18521035
5. Maffulli N, Longo UG, Gougoulias N, Caine D, Denaro V. Sport injuries: a review of outcomes. Br Med Bull. 2011;97:47–80. PMID: 20710023
6. Molnár S, Mensch K, Gáspár K. Wrestling. In: Krutsch W, Mayr H, Musahl V, Della VF, Tscholl P, Jones H, editors. Injury and health risk management in sports. Berlin, Heidelberg: Springer; 2020a. https://doi.org/10.1007/978-3-662-60752-7_86.
7. United World Wrestling, History of Wrestling. [Accessed 2021 July 28]. History of Wrestling & UWW | United World Wrestling
8. United World Wrestling: Medical Regulations (2021) [Accessed 2021 July 28]. title_ENG (uww.org)
9. Molnár SZL, Farkas G, Rögler G, Bacsa P, Péteri L, Gáspár K. Practical medical guide for wrestling competitions - local, regional or younger age competitions. Int J Wrestling Sci. 2014a;4:33–6.
10. Shadgan B, Molnar S, Sikmic S, Chahi A. Wrestling injuries during the 2016 Rio Olympic games. Br J Sports Med. 2017;51:387.
11. Jlid MC, Maffulli N, Elloumi M, Moalla W, Paillard T. Rapid weight loss alters muscular performance and perceived exertion as well as postural control in elite wrestlers. J Sports Med Phys Fitness. 2013;53(6):620–7.
12. Khodaee M, Olewinski L, Shadgan B, Kiningham RR. Rapid weight loss in sports with weight classes. Curr Sports Med Rep. 2015;14(6):435–41. https://doi.org/10.1249/JSR.0000000000000206.
13. Lingor RJ, Olson A. Fluid and diet patterns associated with weight cycling and changes in body composition assessed by continuous monitoring throughout a college wrestling season. J Strength Cond Res. 2010;24(7):1763–72. PMID: 20555285. https://doi.org/10.1519/JSC.0b013e3181db22fb.
14. Shadgan B, Feldman BJ, Jafari S. Wrestling injuries during the 2008 Beijing Olympic Games. Am J Sports Med. 2010;38(9):1870–6. PMID: 20522826
15. Hewett TE, Pasque C, Heyl R, Wroble R. Wrestling injuries. Med Sport Sci. 2005;48:152–78.
16. Thomas RE, Zamanpour K. Injuries in wrestling: systematic review. Phys Sportsmed. 2018;46(2):168–96.

https://doi.org/10.1080/00913847.2018.1445406.
Epub 2018 Mar 9. Review. PubMed PMID: 29484899

17. Myers RJ, Linakis SW, Mello MJ, Linakis JG. Competitive wrestling-related injuries in school aged athletes in U.S. Emergency Departments. West J Emerg Med. 2010;11(5):442–9.

18. Jarret GJ, Orwin JF, Dick RW. Injuries in collegiate wrestling. Am J Sports Med. 1998;26(5):674–80. PubMed PMID: 9784815

19. Yard EE, Collins CL, Dick RW, Comstock RD. An epidemiologic comparison of high school and college wrestling injuries. Am J Sports Med. 2008;36(1):57–64. Epub 2007 Oct 11. PubMed PMID: 17932400

20. Lorish TR, Rizzo TD Jr, Ilstrup DM, Scott SG. Injuries in adolescent and preadolescent boys at two large wrestling tournaments. Am J Sports Med. 1992;20(2):199–202. PubMed PMID: 1558249

21. Mueller FO, Cantu RC. Catastrophic injuries and fatalities in high school and college sports, fall 1982-spring 1988. Med Sci Sports Exerc. 1990;22(6):737–41. https://doi.org/10.1249/00005768-199012000-00001. PMID: 2287249

22. Boden BP, Lin W, Young M, Mueller FO. Catastrophic injuries in wrestlers. Am J Sports Med. 2002;30(6):791–5. PubMed PMID: 12435642

23. Laudermilk J. Catastrophic injuries in junior high school and high school wrestling: a five season study. Chapel Hill: University of North Carolina; 1988. in Hewett TE, Pasque C, Heyl R, Wroble R. Wrestling injuries. Med Sport Sci. 2005;48:152-78. Review. PubMed PMID: 16247257

24. Molnár SZ, Lehto M, Nakajima K, Shadgan B. Guidelines for the Prevention & Management of Strangulation in Olympic Wrestling. United World Wrestling, January 2021. 2021. https://unitedworldwrestling.org/sites/default/files/2021-02/201020_strangulation_in_olympic_wrestling_report_final_version_jan2021.pdf

25. Bruce DA, Schut L, Sutton LN. Brain and cervical spine injuries occurring during organized sports activities in children and adolescents. Prim Care. 1984;11:175–94. in Hewett TE, Pasque C, Heyl R, Wroble R. Wrestling injuries. Med Sport Sci. 2005;48:152-78. Review. PubMed PMID: 16247257

26. Powell JW. National athletic injury/illness reporting system: eye injuries in college wrestling. Int Ophthalmol Clin. 1981;21(4):47–58. PubMed PMID: 7309431

27. Kvittem B, Hardie NA, Roettger M, Conry J. Incidence of orofacial injuries in high school sports. J Public Health Dent. 1998;58(4):288–93. PubMed PMID:10390711

28. Goodman AD, Twomey-Kozak J, DeFroda SF, Owens BD. Epidemiology of shoulder and elbow injuries in National Collegiate Athletic Association wrestlers, 2009-2010 through 2013-2014. Phys Sportsmed. 2018;46(3):361–6. https://doi.org/10.1080/009138 47.2018.1425596. Epub 2018 Jan 18. Erratum in: Phys Sportsmed. 2018 Sep;46(3):vii. PubMed PMID: 29304721

29. Molnár S, Hunya Z, Pavlik A, Bozsik A, Shadgan B, Maffulli N. SLAP lesion and injury of the proximal portion of long head of biceps tendon in elite amateur wrestlers. Indian J Orthop. 2020b;54(3):310–6. https://doi.org/10.1007/s43465-020-00041-6. PMID: 32399150; PMCID: PMC7205930

30. Bak K, Cameron EA, Henderson IJ. Rupture of the pectoralis major: a meta-analysis of 112 cases. Knee Surg Sports Traumatol Arthrosc. 2000;8:113–9.

31. Pavlik A, Csepai D, Berkes I. Surgical treatment of pectoralis major rupture in athletes. Knee Surg Sports Traumatol Arthrosc. 1998;6:129–33.

32. Molnár SZL, Hidas P, Kocsis GY, Rögler G, Balogh P, Farkasházi M, Lang P. Operative elbow injuries among Hungarian elite wrestlers. Case review. Int J Athletic Ther Train. 2014b;19(6):12–6. https://doi.org/10.1123/ijatt.2014-0045.

33. Strauss RH, Lanese RR. Injuries among wrestlers in school and college tournaments. JAMA. 1982;248(16):2016–9. PubMed PMID: 7120629

34. Agel J, Ransone J, Dick R, Oppliger R, Marshall SW. Descriptive epidemiology of collegiate men's wrestling injuries: National Collegiate Athletic Association Injury Surveillance System, 1988-1989 through 2003-2004. J Athl Train. 2007;42(2):303–10. PubMed PMID: 17710180; PubMed Central PMCID: PMC1941299

35. Estwanik JJ, Bergfeld J, Canty T. Report of injuries sustained during the United States Olympic wrestling trials. Am J Sports Med. 1978;6(6):335–40.

36. Lightfoot AJ, McKinley T, Doyle M, Amendola A. ACL tears in collegiate wrestlers: report of six cases in one season. Iowa Orthop J. 2005;25:145–8. PubMed PMID: 16089088; PubMed Central PMCID: PMC1888768

37. Wroble RR, Mysnyk MC, Foster DT, Albright JP. Patterns of knee injuries in wrestling: a six year study. Am J Sports Med. 1986;14(1):55–66. PubMed PMID: 3752347

38. Maffulli N. Making weight: a case study of two elite wrestlers. Br J Sports Med. 1992;26(2):107–10.

39. Mysnyk MC, Wroble RR, Foster DT, Albright JP. Prepatellar bursitis in wrestlers. Am J Sports Med. 1986;14:46–54.